To <u>Dot</u>

With love.

From God

Cherish this book. It contains words flowing from heaven straight through one of God's conduits here on earth. May you also let it flow through you; Nurture it, adding to it the richness God placed in you; and pass it on as you become one of God's Chosen Few.

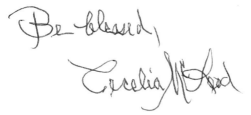

Be blessed,
Cecelia McFord

And God Said To Me...
Do the part of it you
love to do...

Enjoy the Journey

CECELIA MCLEOD

AuthorHouse™
1663 Liberty Drive
Bloomington, IN 47403
www.authorhouse.com
Phone: 1-800-839-8640

First published by AuthorHouse 8/3/2009

ISBN: 978-1-4389-0296-8 (sc)

Printed in the United States of America
Bloomington, Indiana

This book is printed on acid-free paper.

DEDICATION

This series of journals is dedicated first and foremost to God, who changed the path of my life to set me on the journey to do the things He created me to do, and talked with me daily to guide me when my steps faltered.

And to the love of my life, my husband, Lee, who has interspersed tough love and encouragement to take risks, with enough humor and happiness to keep me smiling and fill me with that warm-fuzzy feeling whenever I think back over the 6 years since the stroke we have spent adjusting to my new journey.

To Mother and Daddy (Annie Mae and Allen Green) who encouraged me to always be my best and showed me, by example, how to work side-by-side with my husband to instill values that create a loving family.

To my daughter, Michele, who relieved so much stress, obtaining grants and finding ways to alleviate the caregiving needs for my Mother; and who, along with my son, Mike, applauded each of my accomplishments as I took baby steps in the process of recovering from my stroke.

Also, to my friend, Rita, who encouraged me to publish my conversations with God, written since the stroke, in hopes of helping others understand that they are not alone in their struggles as Stroke Survivors and/or Caregivers.

And to my cousin, Thelma, who believed in and continues to support me in the accomplishment of the three tasks for which God started me on this new journey:

1) The AnnieBand
2) "Enjoy the Journey" plaques
3) Stroke Memories Journals

To my sister, Cat, who replaced Mother and Daddy in believing that I could accomplish anything I truly wanted to do.

To Kim, whose decision to self-publish her book of poetry spurred my decision to stop waiting for others to do for me the things that I could do for myself.

To the caring Doctors and Nurses at Baltimore Washington Medical Center (formerly North Arundel Hospital) and Kernan Hospital who encouraged me to fight this thing.

To James, at Kinkos, who formatted all of the photos in this journal so that you could put a face to the names of some of these wonderful people in my life.

And to all of my prayer partners who prayed with me and for me as we went through the publication process, that this book will touch the lives of all those for whom God intended it.

I am truly blessed.

Preface

A Remarkable Journey

Og Mandino once wrote, "As long as I have something to do, someone to love, and something to hope for, I shall be happy." Well, God has already told me to "Do the part of it I love to do...", and gave me Lee, the love of my life. Now He has shown me the purpose of my life on earth and given me the hope of being able to accomplish it before the end of my time.

You see, God predestined me, before the world began, to do remarkable things. I always knew that I was meant to *make a difference* in this world and used to pray that I would, though, at the time I had no idea how that would happen. God has awakened me before 7 a.m. this morning with the knowledge that I should go to the computer and begin the next task He assigned me while Lee and I were on vacation celebrating my 62nd birthday.

So on this 7th day of April 2006, I am beginning the journey backward, connecting the dots of my life, and fitting the pieces of the puzzle together because God has now given me the gift of discernment. I am excited about this journey because I know that it will reveal ties between events that I never realized existed; events that I thought at the time were coincidental.

These journals are a series of my conversations with God interspersed with what my spirit leads me to feel are His responses to me.

Be with me, Lord; flow through me, helping me to neither add nor take away from the recollection of these events, so that, in the end, a true picture of how You shaped my life will emerge. Thank You Lord. AMEN

Introduction

It's funny how the prospect of writing my *next* book seems almost natural to me even though, in terms of *earth time*, I have not published even the *first* four Stroke Memories Journals nor written the "*Why The Golden Years Are Golden*" book that You inspired while I was on vacation. But I know that those are already done as I wait for *Earth time* to catch up with *God's time.*

At this moment, I have received a denial of disability benefits from Social Security, something that I had banked on to keep us financially stable after I disembarked from Mary Kay, a vehicle that helped me grow into my next role in life. I was used to being able to just sell something almost at will in order to temporarily fill any gap in our cash flow. I guess, by taking away that crutch, God is giving me the opportunity to have life more abundantly by relying on Him to fill all of my needs.

God demonstrated that yesterday when Lee informed me that all the money was gone from the savings account because I had transferred it to pay some overdue bills and now our payment for the new van was due. When I searched our accounts, sure that God would provide an answer on where to get the $512 that was due, I found $589 in my former Mary Kay account! Isn't God AWESOME? He keeps doing things like that and I am so convinced that I can now reassure my sister, who fears that her money is running out, to keep tithing because that is what allowed our Mother's money to last throughout her life with enough leftover to leave an inheritance.

I have received the copyright to the words that God gave to me:

God said to me:

"Do the part of it you love to do.

Don't force it to be what you want it to be,

It will become what it was meant to be.

Love it; Let it flow through you; Nurture it.

Enjoy the Journey.

My cousin, Thelma, overlaid them on the beautiful picture (on the cover of this book) Lee took of me at sunrise on Daytona Beach as I was taking in the awesomeness of the ocean.

I never thought I would be able to take that walk again after the stroke, but I knew I had to go down that morning to meet with God and plead with Him to let Lee live through his pending surgery for prostate cancer. I prayed that He would leave Lee here to walk this journey with me a little while longer. God granted my request.

God inspired me to produce copies of His words to me to share with 144,000 people around the world and to sign and number each one. My first batch was given to some of the friends who have had a powerful impact on my life, such as my Mary Kay Director, Loretta, who was a great mentor to me during my season as a Beauty Consultant.

Those copies were given numbers beginning at 21, because the first 20 numbers were reserved for my family and the most special people in my life; my husband, Lee; daughter, Michele; son, Michael; sister, Cat; brother, Wayne; grandsons, Cameron and Ethan; cousin, Thelma; nephews, Byron and Robert; and special friend, Rita and her family.

The remaining copies will be given to new people that God brings across my new path who need to be encouraged as God gives me a glimpse of what He has in store for them.

Thelma, laughingly said, "Wouldn't it be funny if God had appointed you (me) to select the 144,000 who the Bible showed marching into Heaven; that each of them would, in some way, have received one of these copies?" What an awesome responsibility that would be. That would overwhelm my small mind if I could really take it in, but what an honor it would be!

But even if that is not Your plan, I will proceed with the dropping of the pebble into the lake to start the ripple effect. I will distribute the copies and listen as You call me higher, obeying to the best of my ability.

There was a song that resounded in my spirit (Shekinah Glory's, "Yes"), when I first decided to do this and realized what a commitment I had made now that I had truly said "Yes" to You. When the song reminded me that I might have to give up some relationships and go where I had never gone before, I admit that it scared me to death. But then I prayed that You would allow me to take Lee along on this new journey, even if everyone else was left behind, and You again granted my request. I now know that I will be happy and content in the knowledge that I will always have a human comforter as well as a Heavenly Comforter while I complete my journey here on earth. Thank You, Father, for hearing the cry of one so insignificant in worldly eyes but so significant in Yours.

God has brought many wonderful people to walk this journey with me, some for just a season, but all for the reason of helping me grow into the person He created me to be. These are the most memorable of all those who helped me through this life-changing event:

1. Lee – no greater love has ever been shown by him for me

2. Denise – my first nurse – North Arundel Hospital. Without her, I don't know how I would have made it during that first scary week after the stroke.

3. Kathleen – first nurse—Kernan—ponytail on the side. Tucked me in each night in the beginning, surrounded by pillows to make my back and arm more comfortable. Gave me sleep and pain medication. Stayed past her shift's end to make sure I was taken care of the night when I had chest pains. Quiet smile and nurturing spirit. Reminded me of my sister, Cat. Persevered in getting my new tray sent up when my dinner tray contained foods I shouldn't eat.

4. Doctor Levitt – Doctor In charge of stroke unit at Kernan. Took the time to show compassion and respect. Never looked down at us while we were in wheelchairs. Squatted so that he could talk to us eye to

eye. I later found out that he has Multiple Sclerosis. How uncomfortable it must have been for him to do that, never rushing to complete our discussion.

5. Donna – Black aide at Kernan. Compassionate and caring. Involved in enhancing our stay by doing extra things like organizing the soul food luncheon during Black history month and making sure everyone knew that church services were available on Sundays. Stayed at the hospital 3 days straight during the blizzard of 2003 and gave loving care to us all.

6. Reva – Black nurse at Kernan. Stayed along with Donna during the blizzard. Caring, compassionate. Saw to it that I received the medications needed even when they were just to keep my bowels straight (a stroke affects many muscles including those that control your bowels and even your breathing and swallowing)

7. Jessica – Occupational Therapist – Ker-

nan – taught me how to dress myself one handed. Also how to balance, shower, and go to the bathroom alone. Took me to the gift shop to show me how to shop from the wheelchair and make purchases. Always smiling and encouraging.

8. Debbie – Physical Therapist – Kernan. Showed tough love in instructing and teaching me to try harder to reconnect the brain to the muscles in order to walk. Expected more and discouraged whining.

9. Korron – Psychoanalyst. Encouraged me to talk about my fears and concerns. Got beyond my hard exterior where I could pretend that everything was under control and brought me to a place where I could admit how scared I was that no earthly person was going to be there for me when I ceased to be strong. Who could I talk to, other than God, without putting extra burden on them? I feared that I would no longer be fun to be around, no longer be an encour-

ager, if I let my always-happy façade slip. She let me know that it was all right.

10. Levelle – nurse's aide. Fun loving and helpful.

11. Skevon –nurse's aide. Encouraged and made sure that I got to the Black-history luncheon. Showed Lee and me where to go. Was the first person who was there to give me a hug when I went for my follow-up checkup.

12. Cynthia –fun patient at Kernan. We became dining room buddies. She said that she liked my attitude and that, for her first week at Kernan, she rolled around with her head tied up, and looking like Aunt Jemima. She was so funny. She went home a week before I did and on her last day there, I let her listen to Patti Labelle & T.D. Jakes' "Always There". Tears were streaming down her face. I had Lee make her a copy but she left before I could give it to her. I lost her number and may never see

her again although we had planned to get together.

13. Yvonne – hilarious patient, in constant pain at Kernan.   Short, Black woman, short-blond hair, with a dry sense of humor that would crack you up. Ordered Pepsi at every meal.

14. Ms. Jones (Genevieve?) – Motorized wheel-chair. Nice dining room buddy. Went with me once on an adventure to the cafeteria. Lost her number also. Came to say good-bye the night before I left.

15. Laverne – 50 years old. Came about a week after I did. We talked a lot and laughed together. Hers was the only number I could find after I left the hospital. She had to go back about a month later after for follow-up surgery but seemed in good spirits. We prayed together at the hospital.

16. Lewis – loved coffee. Everyone in our dining-room group always passed him our coffee. Sometimes he would end up with

6 cups. He showed me how to get up the ramp to the cafeteria in my wheelchair and then blocked my fall when I lost momentum and rolled backward. We had a nice talk on the day before he left the hospital in which I tried to encourage him to seek employment in a field he loved.

17. Marshall – patient who always ate all of his food. I admired that because I never had much of an appetite. He was the first person I tried to have a conversation with in the dining room only to find that the stroke had affected his ability to speak. He tried, though, and smiles his understanding. It hurt my heart when I found out that he was being sent to a nursing home when the rest of our group got to go home because his wife couldn't care for him.

18. Virginia – always called her a genteel lady. She was a soft-spoken patient with a gentle smile and always as neat as a pin.

19. Lena – a receptionist at the front desk on

the stroke unit. Lent Lee a TV to play videotapes for me in my room.

20. Janice – nice nurses aide who used to watch star search with Lee and me in the dining room and sing along. Reminded me of a light-skinned Janet Jackson.

21. Fran – nice tiny nurse at Kernan. Took time after work to try to fix the plug connected to my TV so that it would have sound. Didn't give up even after the maintenance men failed to fix it because she saw how frustrated I was when it malfunctioned again for the 6th time.

22. Aree – tiny speech therapist – took the time to stop on her way out on Valentine's Day and put down the flower's from her husband to pull my chart and write up a slip to allow me to have dinner in my room with Lee.

Twenty-two people blessed me with calls, visits, and inspirational gifts and cards, (some as late as 5 months after the stroke) that I will treasure forever.

How blessed I am to have such wonderful friends. It truly surprised me to find out how much people cared.

Who Am I?

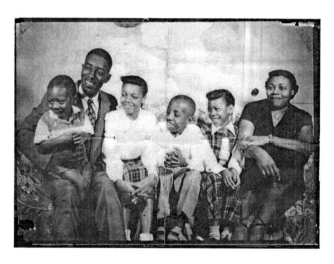

I was the "runt of the litter"; the third child born to my parents within 3 years. My mother delivered me at home, all alone while my father went out on foot (we had no car) to try to find a phone to call the doctor.

It seems that I was always trying to

compensate for my size by proving to everyone that I was special; sometimes by outrunning the other kids in a race (even though I once had an asthma attack before I could finish); climbing higher in the trees (although I once fell when the top branch broke and had the wind knocked out of me); and excelling at school so no one would notice that my self-esteem was low.

I had a bad case of the "*TOO's*"; I was *too* little, *too* skinny (my feet were so skinny that the two sides of my shoes came together when tied, covering the tongue completely); my nose was *too* big; and my legs were so small that my father lovingly called me "sparrow" (he said that only a sparrow had legs that small).

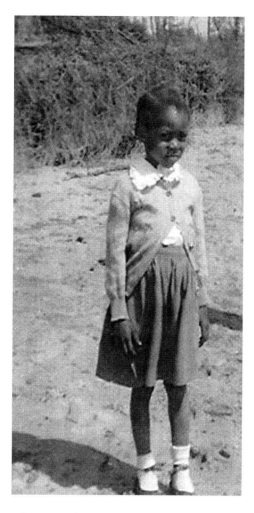

That low self-esteem remained throughout my school and early work years causing me to work harder to achieve. That led to many promotions and a career that started as a secretary, and went through Analyst, Mathematician, Computer Programmer, Designer, Software Engineer, and Engineering Manager; none of which made me feel fulfilled.

It wasn't until I completed a Dale Carnegie course based on the book "How to Win Friends and Influence People" that I began to feel better about myself. The real turning point came though, when I truly got in touch with God and relinquished control to Him (not an easy task for someone who was always afraid to let others see my weakness). But once I *let go and let God* do it, I found that life was no longer the struggle I had made it seem. I began to feel like I was flowing with the stream rather than fighting to stay on top.

My life began to unfold into a lake of gratitude; one in which I could not only float along, but where I could drop a pebble and begin a ripple that would influence the lives of others (some of whom I didn't even know). What a feeling! And the Spirit of God became clearer until I could even hear His voice in my spirit giving me guidance and words of wisdom to live by and eventually to pass on to others.

I started a Corporation, the Christian Computer Community (CCCc) based on a vision He gave me. It provided a safe-learning environment for latch-key kids, taught computer operations and self-esteem enhancement, and children could get help with their homework and a warm meal. It also encouraged Seniors to be loving "joy sharers" as they listened to the children and made history come alive through the sharing of their own stories.

That Corporation, housed in schools and churches, had to be dissolved due to lack of funding before I realized my dream of building our own community. But God's vision still lives through the a program called Watoto Village at my home church and a city-wide program through which Seniors go into the schools to work with the children. Isn't God *Awesome*?

He has grown me so much from that little

girl with low self-esteem into the "God-Powered" woman I am now; much less afraid to take on tasks that I know are from Him. And for those I still fear, I have learned to *"feel the fear and do it anyway."* Thank you Lord. AMEN.

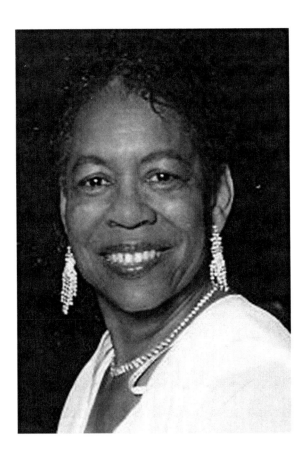

CHAPTER 1-

STROKE MEMORIES

2/3/03

Stroke happened – left side of brain – damage looked about size of a lima bean on the CAT scan. Specialist said later that it was probably due to my high cholesterol level (should be 200 – was over 300 – likely clogged the artery in the brain – blood pressure was also elevated).

I had just come home from the first day of teaching a new Self-Esteem Enhancement course at Mills Parole Elementary School. Things had not gone as smoothly as I had hoped and I pondered on ways to make classes more interesting. Shopping always makes me feel better, so I had stopped at Payless and bought matching suede boots for Mother and me because snow was in the weather forecast.

I had just come back inside after spraying waterproofing on the boots when I felt weakness in my right leg. I thought I'd feel better after I ate (shopping and eating are sure cures for feeling down) and since Lee had prepared dinner, I fixed a plate and brought it to my easy chair. It was then that I felt weakness in my right arm. I told Lee and he thought it was from the spray. Within 15 minutes from the beginning of the episode, the right side of my face went numb and when I tried to call Lee my speech had begun to slur.

I was so scared that I started to cry and have trouble sitting up. I tried to tell Lee to call 911 but my speech was garbled and Lee would not call the ambulance because we lived close to the hospital. Instead, he put socks and slippers on me, backed the van into the driveway, threw me across his shoulder like a sack of potatoes and put me in the van.

I don't know how he managed it, but after arriving at the Emergency Room, he went in and got a wheelchair, and became like an octopus; controlling the chair with one leg, holding the van door open, unstrapping and taking me out of the van, and placing me in the wheelchair (I was dead weight by that time, unable to control any part of my right side).

The receptionist sent me back almost immediately and within ~15 minutes I received a CAT scan. They diagnosed it as a **STROKE**. When I heard the doctor say "stroke", I tried to look behind me to see what old person had walked into the room because I thought he *had* to be talking about someone else. I thought strokes only happened to old people. I really had a lot to learn.

When the doctor who headed the stroke unit told us that, because it was still within a two hour window of the time the stroke had started, I had the option of having a treatment (tPA) that could possibly reverse the effects of the stroke. The drawback was that there was a

6% chance that it could cause bleeding in my brain that they could not stop. In that case, he said, they would have to *"let me die"*. We had only 15 minutes to make the decision and tried unsuccessfully to reach my Primary Care Physician for advice. Needless to say, we did not take that option.

I truly believe that God had a reason for allowing this stroke to happen. Even though I ate right and walked 1 to 3 miles almost daily, and neither smoked nor drank, I believe that God sometimes has to slow us down enough to allow us to make the turn on our life's path to put us on the journey toward the thing He created us to do.

Other immediate effects of the stroke included:

1. Shortness of breath – weakened muscle under diaphragm

2. Tiredness when trying to talk

3. Inability to swallow without thinking it through

4. Lack of balance – stayed in bed most of the five days at North Arundel Hospital except during times of therapy

5. Tongue wasn't working properly. Months later, the right side of my tongue was still not back to normal.

6. The need to cry – tears were always just below the surface even though I didn't exactly feel sad. I just never found a time when I could cry without fear of upsetting someone. I had always been the person with all the joy and positive outlook and now I just had the overwhelming need to just have one good cry. Denise let me know that it was alright.

Denise was my nurse at North Arundel Hospital and the most loving, caring person I could have met. I don't know how I would have made it through those first trying days without her. She not only gave excellent nursing care but offered words of consolation and hope, a willing ear, a shoulder to cry on, and even a time alone to cry when that was what I needed most. Right in the middle of that cry, the doctor came in and looked so helpless when he saw my tear-stained face.

Denise gave me hugs and humor, enough semi-tough love to encourage me to start fighting this thing, and even came to see me on her day off because it was the day I was being discharged to go to the rehab hospital. I had not been allowed to go to the bathroom – only allowed to use bedpans which kept spilling when the aides removed them, wetting my bed causing them to have to roll me over to change it- a humiliating experience. Then, to add insult to injury, my bowels locked up.

Denise gave me a laxative and sat me on a commode. What blessed relief it was to have a bowel movement before going off to a strange place. Denise even gave follow-up calls to me at Kernan and at home. She truly exemplifies what a nurse should be.

Shipping Out and Arrival at Kernan Rehab Hospital

I was ready to go long before the ambulance crew who were supposed to drive me finally located my room. I was a little leery about traveling with snow and slick spots on the ground, but we arrived safely at Kernan at about 7:30p.m. on Friday, February 7, 2003, the beginning of a life-changing month.

I don't recall a lot about that night except that Lee met us at the hospital. A wonderful nurse named Kathleen was assigned to me that night and she and an aide named Marge made me feel welcome. Kathleen tucked pillows around me to support my weak arm and tried to make me comfortable in every way she knew how. I didn't realize then just how much I would come to depend on her in the next month. Thank you God for all those you sent to help make this experience as pleasant as possible. I still look back on it with a feeling of warmth in my heart.

When I look back on that time years later, these are the memories that stand out:

1. A loving rehabilitation "boot camp" with our therapy schedules posted on our doors every morning. We were assisted in washing and dressing early each morning and we met in the dining room for breakfast. I was proud to be able to propel my wheelchair with one foot at a pretty good clip. I realized later how strange I must have looked when I heard someone say I was moving like a crab ☺ .But that didn't matter because I could get to the place I was heading faster than most of the others.

2. Our table in the dining room was the fun table and we laughed a lot while trying not to choke on our food and drinks, lest the

nurses feel they needed to add (the dreaded) thickener to our drinks. Sometimes when Lee was visiting, he would make me laugh and choke and then threaten to call a nurse to add thickener.

3. I would welcome the "newbies" into the dining room because I realized how scary the situation must be for those who did not have outgoing personalities. I encouraged the last newbie to carry on this practice after I left.

4. One of the most humiliating things that happened to me was to be dependent on the nurses to answer my call to take me to the bathroom when I needed to go.

I requested a laxative because the muscles that control my bowels had not yet normalized. However, when I felt I needed to go, I once had to wait 45 minutes for a nurse to respond. I held it in, propelled myself around to the front desk, and was in tears by the time I reached Dr. Levitt, who headed up the Stroke Unit. After

I (almost incoherently) sobbed out the story, he had a nurse take me into the nearest bathroom. By that time, my bowels (that never functioned in front of an audience) completely locked up because the nurse was afraid to leave me alone in the bathroom. I finally convinced her to help me onto the toilet and stand outside the room.

Every situation has a good side, though, and this one made me even more determined to learn to go to the bathroom alone. I was thinking the other day of the ritual I had to go through at the hospital just to get to the bathroom:

1. pulling myself up with the noisy bed control

2. getting my shoes on for traction without losing my balance

3. getting in the wheelchair without falling

4. scooting the chair out without getting it caught in the curtain that separated the room

5. opening the bathroom door

6. scooting hard enough with one foot to get

over the bump at the entrance to the bath-room

7. turning the chair around and scooting it back out far enough to close the door

8. positioning the chair between the rails and balancing myself on one foot with one hand to drop my pajamas and use the bathroom.

9. Hoping the toilet paper was wound around the rail enough for me to reach

10. balancing to pull up my pajamas

11. getting back into the chair

12. reversing the whole process to get back into bed.

That consumed most of an hour. But it was worth it, because they were my first steps toward regaining my independence.

3/2/03

Lee came to Kernan on the first beautiful, sunny day since the snow. He appeared just after church service and asked if I would like to go outside. I was delighted at the prospect of being out and he rolled my wheelchair to the van. I thought it was to get away from the smokers at the door. Then he asked how I would like to go for a ride. I was thrilled and felt like a kid sneaking out of school. Once I was in the van, he asked how I would like to go home for awhile. I was so excited!

I kept trying to drink in the sights that had seemed so ordinary to me only a month ago. Traffic jams on the beltway, and piles of dirty snow. Blue skies had never looked so beautiful! I know how a prisoner must feel after being released for the first time. It was excitement mixed with a little trepidation. I had left the protected environment of Kernan where doctors and nurses were around to tend to my every need and bars were there to catch me if I stumbled. Would I be able to cry if the mood struck me at home or would I have to go back to being a superwoman?

I had gotten used to meals always ready and

waiting and my meds on time. Would I be a burden on Lee not being able to do for myself? Would the lack of handicap equipment at home cause me to hurt myself, and did I want to appear helpless in Lee's eyes? All these questions were in my mind but for no reason. Lee had planned the whole Sunday and swore everyone, even the doctors and nurses, to secrecy.

Mike and Heather along with Michele, Everett and the boys came and we had dinner and dessert and a wonderful visit before Lee took me back. It was a memorable day but I was secretly glad to go back to what had become my "safe haven".

3/4/03 -- Coming Home

The therapists and doctor agreed that I had made such progress that I could choose to go home a day early if I desired. A little fearful but excited, I asked Lee to pick me up. I spent most of my time the day before packing up what I could but Lee told me he would take care of it. Before checking out, several therapists, nurses and aides came to say goodbye. Even Mrs. Jones and Lavern, good friends I had made during my stay at rehab, came to my room. I will miss them but I know that I will probably recuperate more quickly at home.

When I arrived home, Lee had placed the single rose that Loretta had brought to the hospital in the bathroom above my makeup case. He put a basket on the counter containing the toiletries that I would need. He laid out my medications in a daily-dosage container and made up my bed in the spare room when I tossed and turned and found that I could not sleep comfortably in our waterbed.

Lee arranged pillows in the spare room bed to support my weak arm and to prop up my head. He stayed in the room until I was tucked in and parked my wheelchair beside the bed so that I could easily reach it. Then he would kiss me good night. He placed a two-way transmitter beside my bed on the chair where he also put a box of tissues and my water bottle. I feel so loved and protected.

I had looked forward to seeing the Queen Latifa/Steve Martin movie ever since I had first heard it advertised. I never dreamed that I would be able to get out and see it after all this new drama. But Lee surprised me 3 days after I got home by taking me out on date night, rolling my wheelchair onto the elevator at Arundel Mills and settling me on the upper level of the theatre to see that movie. What a wonderful surprise! He sat protectively close beside me and I truly enjoyed myself. Isn't it funny how things you have taken for granted before can seem so very special when you haven't done them for awhile?

Lee was wonderful, taking me out to lunch after therapy, making sure I remembered to take my medication, and even finding a small bottle in which to carry my evening meds if we were going to be out. If we ever did not have the meds with us, he mixed them with applesauce and gave them to me in a cup when we got home. We watched American idol and Star Search together and he found different desserts to surprise me with most nights. He recorded programs so that I would be entertained whenever I ate.

He sets my food and hot tea on the small table that he had purchased shortly before I had the stroke, and gives me a variety of balanced meals everyday. When I felt the need for a good soaking, he helped me get into the tub and get settled. At first I was a little shy about having him see me naked even though we had often showered together before. It just seems different when he is dressed and I am not. I soon got over it and he even had to help me get out of the tub by climbing in and taking my hands to lift me. How special he makes me feel.

Yesterday was a beautiful Spring-like day with temperatures in the 70's. Lee had back-to-back weddings because Neal, Mike's friend, was getting married at 6:00 in the evening. Mother decided to "Mommy-sit" me during the day and Michele came in the evening. It seems so odd to have people taking care of me. But it's like a passage in the book Paulette Stallings sent—"God would prefer an occasional limp rather than a perpetual strut". This told me that I don't have to pretend that things are just right all the time. I used to think that the admission that things weren't going smoothly for me was a sign of weakness, fallibility, and a betrayal to my gift of joy. I felt ungrateful and, if I gave in to those feelings, that I had chosen to be unhappy.

I see life as a series of choices and I felt much better in choosing to be happy. Unfortunately, this did not free everyone around me to show their true feelings and kept me from seeing the giving, caring nature that others possessed. I am seeing that now and it blows my mind. It also allowed me to take off the rose-colored glasses and stop making excuses for Tina, the one person whom I called my best friend.

For a long time, I made excuses for her calling only when she needed something and my having to be the one who always initiated the makeup after we had a disagreement. After rescuing her and being there for her so many times and even encouraging her to write a book, lending her the typewriter and showing her how to save files on the computer, she dedicated her first book to my friends Shirley and Gwen because they took her for a haircut and lunch. But the final wake-up call came after I called her from the hospital and told her about my stroke and she made no effort to get in touch with anyone for the month I was hospitalized to inquire about me.

When I got home and checked my email, the note from her said that she expected to hear more from me but she "guessed that *she* wasn't important enough". That still hurts even now, that she would even make *my* stroke "*about her*". Sometimes, as my father used to say, I guess You have to "hit us with a 2x4", Lord, to drive a point home. They say that, if being around a person makes you feel worse, then stay away from that person. I have learned my lesson. Thank you Lord.

But I've gained so many positive insights about the people who surround me with love that it seems like you are saying that if I remove one negative force from my life, you will flood me with the blessings of so many others too numerous to count. Rita, my daughter's Mother-in-law and my good friend, gave me some words of wisdom that helped me get over the bitterness and let it go. She said "Sometimes, the best thing you can do for a person who doesn't have your best interest at

heart is just to pray for them and let them go."
And I did.

Thank you for the special blessing of Lee,
Lord. From the day I entered the hospital,
he was there every morning, bringing me
whatever I needed and lending moral support.
He even brought me a portable CD player and
headsets that allowed me to shut out hospital
noises when I so badly needed peace and rest.
He brought me the two CDs. One was "God's
Leading Ladies" on which Patti Labelle and
T.D. Jakes sang "Always There". Little did
I realize when I fell in love with that song
months before that those words would be such
a comfort to me later. But you knew, didn't you
Lord? Just like You knew that the words from
Isaiah 41:10 ("*Fear thou not, for I am with thee,
be not dismayed for I am thy God." I will comfort
thee, yea, I will help thee; yea, I will uphold thee
with the right hand of my righteousness*") would
shore me up when I needed them most. Lee
also brought me the CD that he created and
labeled "Quiet Times" that soothed me to sleep

when I needed it.

He even came to Kernan through the deep snow to bring me food whenever I didn't like what they served. He picked up my dirty clothes every time he came and returned them clean and folded the next day. He brought me treats and videotaped segments of shows we could watch together on the big screen television.

On Valentine's Day, Lee made me a beautiful Valentine's poster-board card that must have taken all day. It had the Olan Mills portrait of the of us and the kids; a picture of Everett & Michele dancing; a picture of Mike and Heather; one of our grandsons, Cameron and Ethan; pictures taken with the video camera of my prayer room, the screen room, the snowy view out back; the shot of both sides of the family taken at his retirement party; a picture of Mother; and a picture of him. He also bought me beautiful sets of undies and a gold box of Godiva chocolate-covered cherries. He picked out a wonderful card that told me that he couldn't imagine life without me by his side.

We watched videos together and ended the night with one of the most special things he had begun again-- kissing me every time we parted. They were not long passionate kisses like before but a kiss that said "I love you". I didn't realize how much I had missed the feel of his lips. Now, I long to feel him hold me again but I think he's afraid to break me. He said one time in the hospital that he couldn't give me a massage because he might throw me into cardiac arrest.

It didn't help that I got chest pains one night at Kernan and Lee came up in the middle of the night, even though he was on medication for an infected, painful tooth. What love! One day there was a Black heritage luncheon and Lee surprised me by even showing up to take me there.

I had a bad episode one day after the doctors came and gave me 2 cortisone shots in my shoulder to alleviate pain from a subluxation I had caused by trying too hard to make my affected arm stretch (exercising the old "no pain-no gain" theory). I was glad Lee was there but I started feeling dizzy right after the shots, scaring me and causing me to cry, and I wanted to get on the bed.

Lee kept trying to get me to say what was wrong, but by now I was trying not to cry and couldn't talk. He ran to get the doctor and everybody kept asking me what was wrong. I was surrounded by people but I couldn't understand why Lee was standing in the doorway instead of holding me to make it better. I got mad at him and screamed at him to make it stop but he just stood there and let the doctors do their work.

I felt so alone. I don't think he realizes that sometimes I don't expect him to fix a problem, I just need him to hold my hand and assure me that he is there with me and I don't have to face this by myself; that he understands what I'm going through and we'll get through this together.

I try to be the strong one for the family but

it's scary to wonder who, besides God, will be there for me if I let my true weakness show. Now I know. You have surrounded me with all of these people whose lives I have touched, who I didn't think could make it without my holding their hand, or who didn't really care. And now here they are. Showing and telling me what an impact I have made on their lives. They make me feel so special and so grateful.

But they must have seen You, through me, because my motives were not always directed outside of myself. But You saw the good and made that the focal point, to outshine all my human misdirection. Thank you Lord for ordering my steps.

3/26/03 – My Birthday

The forecast said that this was supposed to be the worst day this week with clouds and rain all day but again you proved that I'm one of your favorite people. I awoke to sunny, blue skies and birds singing. I had said that I wanted to make this a "pamper me" day with the hairdresser, nail salon, and a massage. When I awoke, however, I pictured feeding seagulls by the water and satisfying my craving for a quesadilla. I didn't mention this but just started my day with a nice, leisurely shower and dressed in a sunny, yellow jogging suit.

As soon as I came out of the bathroom, Lee asked if I would like to go out to breakfast. We ended up at the Inner Harbor where the weather was beautiful and we found an ideal parking spot. We went to a Tex-Mex restaurant where

I had a quesadilla out on the deck overlooking the harbor. We strolled awhile with Lee walking beside me pushing the wheelchair and then visited a Christmas shop where I saw the cutest mouse display and Lee told me to pick out two. I chose one that he pointed out with a mouse bursting out of a flowerpot surrounded by sunflowers and smiling at a bluebird. The other was a boy and girl mouse standing under a red umbrella with clear, heart shaped raindrops falling from it.

As if that wasn't enough, Lee had put corn chips from the restaurant in a napkin and took me near the water where I fed the seagulls. Then we went in the pavilion where I got a cone of orange sherbet and he got cookies. We got back in the van just before the raindrops started to fall. Thank you Father. And you weren't finished yet. Loretta and Irie showed up at my door after we had a nap, filled my client's order for delivery, and took my preferred customer list to prepare a letter for a Mary Kay $1000 day.

Lee offered to take me out for dinner (which I postponed until tomorrow) and baked special chocolate brownies that tasted like Easter chocolate. How blessed I am. Mother called and said she had some clotting and bleeding after dialysis and some palpitations after she got home. She had ignored the advice of the dialysis tech to go to the hospital. Thank you for letting her listen to me. She is now safely admitted in North Arundel Hospital after Thelma called 9-1-1 and Lee went up to let them in. What a birthday! Thanks for blessing me Lord and thanks so much for the love of Lee.

3/27/03

It was a beautiful, sunny, near-70-degree day and I just had to get outside. I left Lee a note and made my way, with shakey steps, down to the foyer, out the front door, and around to the back yard. It was marvelous! I sat on the chest where we store birdseed and watched the birds and squirrels play. I took my camera and even managed to take some pictures left-handed. The flowering crabapple tree was in bloom in the front yard so I took pictures of it as well.

Then I was really feeling my oats so I went inside, made and ate some raisin toast and juice for breakfast, and then Lee set up the hose while I made my way, backward, down the back steps and proceeded to clean the three lawn chairs (Lee pulled out the chaise and I got the other two). I was quite proud of myself when I finished. I came back in, prepared to spend the rest of the day out on the porch alone because Lee had a wedding to tape.

But God rewarded my perseverance by having Mother call and invite me out to dinner. We had dinner at Golden Corral and had a good time. Who would have believed that my 82-year-old Mother would be picking me up and dropping me at the door of a restaurant while she found a parking space? Chances sure do go around.

4/20/03 - EASTER

Michele invited us down for dinner and to celebrate Rita's birthday which will be next week. I went to church with Mother and broke down when they sang "God is". I recovered nicely. I went without my chair. I have gone without it for about 2 weeks now, using just my brace and cane. Michele had dyed extra eggs for Mother and me and surprised us with baskets for her, Lee and me.

We had a really nice time and the boys were delightful. I was glad to be able to make a spa basket for Rita and Mike made her two CDs and Lee did a wonderful CD of "Quiet Times" selections he had given to me that soothed me at the hospital. He made a label with a picture of the boys on it. He had already given her the wonderful CD "God's Leading Ladies" by T.D.

Jakes and Patti Labelle.

4/21/03

Lee took me for a ride and we ended up in Towson after seeing beautiful flowering bushes along the way. We decided to take in a movie. I felt like a schoolgirl playing hooky. I really don't ever remember going to the movies on Monday night. We went to the newer theatre there at my suggestion but I really didn't realize that it was only accessible by escalator. I was scared to get on but Lee reassured me that he wouldn't let me fall and he didn't (even though he was only holding the back of my jacket with 2 fingers). I felt like I had overcome another major hurdle when I had gone up and down that escalator. Thank you God for Lee who keeps encouraging me to step out of my comfort zone and take risks.

4/28/03- A Minor Breakthrough

Some gripping ability in my right hand! I was doing some stretching and found that I could grip the bedrail in the spare room for 15 seconds. I also made fish & chips and broccoli for dinner. After cleaning out my built-in this morning, my legs and arm started to feel heavy again.

And I finally got a decent night's sleep! I've had many sleepless nights during which I tried sleeping in the recliner, the massage chair, and a combination of both. It ultimately required pain pills and a cortisone shot in the hip to give me some relief. Thank you, Jesus.

And I want to give you special thanks for my friend, Rita, who kept me company via email during the many nights that I couldn't sleep. It was always a comfort to be able to share my thoughts, fears, and triumphs with her and read her enthusiastic caring responses. This was a tremendous help, especially in the first few months following the stroke when speaking was not a comfortable option.

5\5\03

I washed clothes for the first time since the stroke. After sorting them into bundles, Lee took them downstairs for me. I felt so proud that I could do that again.

5/7/03

Lee was working hard all day, doing the lawn and trying to finish up the videos he had promised people he'd have for them by Mother's day. I heated dinner –leftover fish—and made cornbread and succotash. I never thought I could feel so proud cooking.

Lee and I watch American idol and Star Search together, sitting on our lounge chairs.

Sometimes in the afternoon we will even take a nap at the same time. It is good to awaken and watch him sleeping across from me. He thinks up something inviting and healthy for each meal and seems to sense when my muscles have given out for the day. The other evening, he offered me strawberry yogurt and added fresh strawberries that he had cut up and sweetened. I don't know why he loves me so much but I thank God that he does.

5/9/03

I rode with Lee to Monkton, MD to attend a rehearsal for a wedding he is doing tomorrow. The scenery was beautiful. Afterwards, we came back down here for a movie and I opted to leave my chair in the van. I am a little slow but he walked with me. He teased me as I slowly made my way up the steps, saying that, "If there was a fire, I was on my own" ☺. He keeps everything light and humorous so that I don't take myself too seriously. I hope that he realizes just how much more pleasant he has made this experience for me. When I look back on it in years to come, I'm sure it will be with a feeling of warmth and love.

5/17/03

Today Mike took me out to lunch at the Olive Tree. He had promised this as a part of my birthday gift. We had a wonderful lunch, laughing and talking and then he suggested that, if I didn't have other plans, he would take me for a ride to see some fabulous new homes along the back roads where he rides his motorcycle. It was lovely; winding country roads lined with tall trees and yards brimming with all colors of spring flowers. Then it was home again where I was free to dress in my soft, flannel jammies and settle in the easy chair for a short nap.

Lee and his brother, Jay, were off doing a wedding and I just decided to have leftover Chinese food for dinner and write an entry in this journal while listening to the T.D. Jakes CD. It's funny how that CD still brings back pleasant memories of Kernan. God was good enough to surround me with wonderful loving people since the stroke so the memories will always fill me with warmth.

It is sad to think of Essie in my Mary Kay unit who has been hospitalized again since her stroke, and Laverne Caison, who I met at Kernan, is back in the hospital after having another operation. I thank God that I am recuperating and pray that I will not have to repeat the experience. It was bearable the first time but to do it again would seem like starting over from square one. I know God would be with me but I pray I that I have accomplished the thing the stroke needed me to accomplish.

One major accomplishment was to show Lee and Linda why they needed blood pressure medicine. If it saved their lives, I am grateful to have gone through this experience. Thank you Lord for using me.

5/21/03

Today I feel your urgings to have me begin my daily entries to my journal once again. This time, they will all be online and done again first thing in the morning. It's funny, now when I feel my weakest, Lee is responding totally opposite than what I expected. I always thought that he stayed away from people who seem dependent and that he was attracted to my strong will and independence. I hear you telling me that it appeared so because that was the time when I seemed most content.

People like to feel needed. I guess that I am seeing that also in the rest of my friends and family. Help me to appreciate that without taking advantage of it. Help me to still try to do things myself before seeking help but not be too proud to ask for it when necessary. Help me to step out knowing that I can do all things through You as long as I have faith to know that you won't let me fall.

Yesterday, I found out that I still have a sore

spot in my feelings when I was trying to clean the lounge chair cushions and something didn't go right. Lee asked me why I always tried to make things so hard. That started tears that I couldn't seem to stop for about half an hour. Didn't he realize that it *was* hard and it wouldn't be if all my limbs would just work as they were supposed to? Even now, it still makes the tears flow. I know that he didn't mean to hurt my feelings and that he felt badly about making me cry.

He did the right thing by not mentioning my tears but just went and got some other stuff to help me clean and then worked close by in the yard where he could keep an eye out for me. He later made some small talk about things he was doing and even brought out the wicker sofa with its brightly-colored cushions from under the deck for me to brush off. That cheered me and I sat on it later and had lunch in front of the hibiscus bushes that Lee had placed around the edge of the patio. Thank you for sending the birds to cheer me.

I'm still enjoying the time I'm spending with Lee, eating fresh fruit –pineapple, strawberries, and cantaloupe—that he bought at giant and cut up into bite-sized pieces. He even offered me that part of the pineapple skin that had a lot of fruit still on it—oh, was it sweet! Then we both lounged in our chairs to watch American Idol together after having dinner of grilled fresh salmon, broccoli and mashed potatoes. I was even able to wash the pots and start the dishwasher before sitting down for the evening.

I thank you for letting me sometimes have more energy left to be of help in the evenings. Please help me to keep listening to my body, attempting to do things when I can but not being discouraged when I can't. Thank you for the strength and faith that lets me go up and down the back steps and across the yard now. Today, I will attempt to get all of our bills online so that they may be easily paid. Bless me Lord so that I may be a blessing. AMEN

5/22/03

Lord I thank you for this new day and for a good night's sleep last night. Yesterday when I felt sluggish, I thank you for letting me have the wisdom to stop and rest. Lee and I enjoyed the time together sitting down to watch the finals of American Idol after I had done dishes and folded clothes. It is good to know that I can now make myself take on small tasks with the determination to finish them and then find that You give me the strength I need.

Thank you for giving me the perseverance to set up the bill payer program even though Lee and I differ in opinion of how much detail is needed before I take it over. Thank you for letting us disagree and still be on friendly terms later.

Thanks for the reminder through Luther Van Dross' stroke of just how blessed I really am. A person never knows whose life may be influenced by his circumstances. That causes me to wonder just how many lives I have touched through mine. Thank you, Lord, for using me.

The Mary Kay Director, Pam, wrote that people are watching to see how I handle this. Please let me be a positive example of your love. Thank you Lord. AMEN

5/24/03

Thank you God for this new day. I don't feel that it's a breakthrough day but I never know just what blessings you have in store for me. Byron is gone to Myrtle Beach and called Mother to say they arrived safely. Thank you for bringing him into Mother's life on a daily basis. I know that it's only temporary but it is doing so much to add pleasure to her life, to once again have someone to talk to and someone to watch over her.

Mike and Heather are gone to California with friends for a leisurely trip up the coast. Thank you for watching over them and giving them the means and desire to travel at will.

Thanks for the dinner out with Lee last night

where we talked about the sports events that were on the TV at the Glory Days restaurant. It is truly a joy spending this much time with him. This morning I was up early enough to hear Lee Michaels' "Spiritual Vitamin" and enjoy a good stretch in the spare room. It's funny how these little pleasures can be so significant. I'm really looking forward to Date Night tonight when Lee and I will get to see "Bruce Almighty". Life is good and I'm continuing to improve. Thank you Lord. AMEN

P.S. Today, I'm going to start writing thank you notes to all the friends who remembered me throughout this growth experience. If they felt that it was never too late to send cards and gifts, I feel that it is never too late to say "thank you".

When Lee and I went to the movies, he decided I should take the wheelchair even though I have not used it for over a month. He didn't want me to have to walk long distances. I told him that I was going to miss his walking next to me so protectively when we return the chair next week. However, I am grateful for the progress. Thank you Lord.

5/27/03

Hooray! Progress! Today I was able to hold the phone between the pointer finger and thumb of my right hand and carry it from the living room to the spare room and back twice before dropping it. I even swung my arm. I was so proud I showed Lee. Thank you Lord. You know when I am getting a bit discouraged and you give me a little hope to build on.

We went to Lee's second cousin's graduation party on Sunday and a cookout at Becky's house yesterday, so our holiday weekend was pretty full. Everyone is still being helpful; Linda loading my plate and Paula looking after my needs at the cookout. I am truly blessed.

I was lying in bed thinking this morning of the folks who have to fend for themselves and how hard it must be to get to therapy and doctor's appointments, not to mention purchasing, hauling and cooking food and remembering all the new medicines. Add to this the fear of taking unsure steps knowing that you may fall and have people misunderstand your situation.

I have been blessed to not only have people ready and willing to care for my needs but also there to see that most of my wants are taken care of. I am able to go out for entertainment and socialization and hugged and kissed to made to feel special. To top it off, you show your delight in me by sending, this morning, my first chipmunk of Spring, a Blue Jay, a Cardinal, 3 squirrels, and 2 yellow finches to delight me as they fed at the overflowing birdfeeders that Lee filled. So Lord, help me not to complain or feel slighted when I don't get that backrub that I would like or when Lee seems a little reluctant to fulfill one of my requests. Help me to let him know just how grateful I am to have him without embarrassing him.

Thank you for Michele's helpfulness as she took Mother to the eye doctor this morning, and please let whatever is causing Mother to have short memory losses to be corrected soon. I know that the issue of my crooked fingers is being resolved although that should be the least of my worries now.

Help me to give back, Lord. I want to get involved by teaching others some lessons I have learned but have not yet figured a way to get there without putting extra work on Lee. I know it will come to me.

6/12/03

Today I had the last Physical Therapy session that the insurance would cover. The leg is stronger now and I am able to walk forward when I go down the front and back stairs. The arm can sometimes carry things and I'm able to lift it back down from overhead when I'm lying flat on my back, though not yet with control.

I contacted the Department of Recs and Parks to see if I could still get paid for the 2 days I spent in planning and teaching the "Self-Esteem Enhancement" class before the stroke.

I was surprised to find that they were not only willing to pay for that, but also for the time I spent planning for the Etiquette classes. They even asked if I would be willing to come back to teach again! I told them that I would as soon as I was able to drive. I don't want to be dependent on someone else for transportation.

I also spoke to a person about designing and teaching a course in life skills for those with disabilities. She asked me to send her a course outline that she could look it over because they had nothing like it, thus far. The description just flowed through my fingers and I submitted it within a week. I'm beginning to feel stirrings of independence.

Lee reminded me last Friday that we still need money for Disney and he asked if I was still doing Mary Kay. I told him that I was but only when people called me. He asked me if I called them anymore. It's funny; he seems to want me to do the things that he gave negative feedback for before. When I used to give out business cards freely, have people over for facials, spend a lot of phone time calling potential clients, and talking "too loudly and too much", I felt negative vibes. Now that I can't speak loudly or as much and have ceased giving out cards, he is asking about it. Loretta must be right when she says that I should just be myself and do whatever comes naturally.

Mother drove me across town to deliver product to one of the Seniors at Wyman House today. We were caught in a horrendous downpour with wind, thunder, and lightning. We kept going even though water was flooding the streets because we were caught up in traffic with no good way to turn back. We even had people blowing and going around us as we tried to find a safe place to pull over. You protected us and even stopped the storm long enough for us to park in front of the door of the building. You held back the rain long enough for me to go inside, make my delivery, and get back in the car and even allowed the sun to peek through to show us that it was alright to go home safely. Thank you God.

I am going to seriously tackle the task of sending out thank you notes to all who remembered me in my hour of need. I will do this before the passion that I felt lessens and the gratitude fails to truly show through. Please be with me Lord lest I forget for one moment just how much it meant to be remembered.

I am in a dilemma now because I planned to modify the note I wrote to Lee about how much his care has meant to me and put it in his Father's day card. But I can't find the file. I am up at 5 a.m. and I'm concerned about not having a Father's day gift for him even though he bought an expensive digital camera and said that it was a Mother's Day and Father's Day gift. Somehow, I wanted to get him something to show him just how much he means to me. I guess I'll just give him the stepping stones he wanted for the backyard if Michele can find them and try to show him I care with my everyday actions.

6/26/03

Yesterday I cried again – frustration, anger, helplessness—all three. My right arm and hand are still not working properly and I am really trying to do things for myself. I was attempting to cut off some pieces of cantaloupe while Lee was out mowing the lawn. I was trying to be careful because the knife was sharp and I didn't want to injure myself again (I was already scheduled to go for x-rays today to evaluate injury to my right toe and left thumb from my most recent fall).

Lee had said before that I was "too scared" and I was determined that I would prove him wrong. Anyway, I tried every way I could to hold the cantaloupe still with the weak hand while trying to cut it with the left but it kept slipping. After about 15 frustrating minutes, Lee came in and seeing me struggling for about 5 minutes more, asked if I needed help with it. I just lost it and sobbed against the refrigerator, ashamed and embarrassed that I still could not complete a task so simple.

I went to the bathroom to try to recover my composure and when I felt I had gotten myself together, came out and found that he had cut the cantaloupe and gone out to the porch. He has learned that it is best in those situations to just leave me alone to work it out. I gathered my food as I had intended and went down to the patio to eat it and exercise. I had had such determination to make progress that morning but Satan influenced my mind and caused it to look like a setback. I cried a few more tears out on the lounge chair before looking up through the leaves above me to see the beautiful blue skies, the yellow and black finches, the large red hibiscus bloom, and the tiny chipmunk that You sent to delight me. That was Your way of reminding me that it is alright to cry.

I lowered the back of my lounge chair and began to exercise my arms and legs just as I had planned. Satan is always looking for signs of weakness and uses the opportunity to make you doubt yourself and your abilities. I just need to remember not to buy into it. I have choices. Thank you, God, that I also know You, who always delight in me and send things to cheer me so that I am not down too long.

Lee took Mother, Aunt Liz, Linda, Weebie, and I out to Sham Denai's, a waffle and chicken place, for a delightful dinner. Tuesday night, when I had spent a tiresome day and just slept through dinner, he took me up the street to a new ice cream place where we sat out on a bench and ate ice cream on a warm, summer night. Sunday, he took me to the new Outback Steak House for dinner. He is really a blessing in my newly-discovered mission to spread joy. Please, God, help me to start with him because he adds such joy to my life.

I am continuing to get cards and well wishes from people. Different members of my church (New Psalmist Baptist) have sent cards every week since they learned of the stroke. Michelle and I have started attending Mary Kay meetings again and I even had a self-invited guest to come as a model last Monday (Vikki Jones). My Mary Kay team members have continued working their businesses to the point where I am still a Team Leader. I guess it just shows that I don't have to beg or coerce people to do what they want to do.

I have still not decided what I want to do with my Mary Kay career as far as advancement goes, but I know that I will share the testimony of how good it is to have a business that will continue to at least provide me with spending money and tithes even when I can't work it. It also provides a support system and sisterhood that is hard to find elsewhere.

Loretta and Irie have been right there for me with encouragement and suggestions to get me back on my feet without pushing. I think that it is Loretta's newly-found faith that is helping her really be there for me and Satan is trying to defeat our unit on every hand. We are not giving up, though, because we know who has our back.

I started making this entry at about 3:30 this morning after lying in the dark for about an hour with thoughts of the deformity and uselessness of this right hand. However, in looking at it in the light, I find that it is not deformed at all, but there is just a slight bend to my little finger. My job is just to pray over it and dedicate its use to God and He will strenghthen it to do his work. I feel better already.

I have been beating myself up for neglecting to send thank you notes to all who have been so thoughtful with their gifts during this time. But I now am taking heed to something you have been whispering in my ear every time I thought of it…"*Pass it on*" is what you are saying. What greater "thank you" could I say than to do for others what your children have done for me? Thank you Lord. I think I'll go back to bed and snuggle up with Lee now. Good night.

6/27/03

Awake at 4:35 a.m. – tried to sleep almost flat as was advised in the stroke magazine. My arm muscles are very tight. I woke up thinking about bills that I pre-authorized twice as I try to get my entries in the Bill-payer program straightened out. I decided to get up and make list to check and also decided to look up a local Stroke Support group.

I am reluctant about joining a Stroke Support group because I'm afraid that it might put me in the mindset of being permanently in the "sick or disabled" instead of the "normal" group. Am I in denial about my new limitations? The arm hanging helplessly at my side or drawing up into a "stroke appearance" bothers me more than I admit. I try to look around at the displays or even the ceiling while I am walking from the movies to meet Lee at the curb and try to pretend that it doesn't bother me to walk like I'm "handicapped".

I never realized that I had a prejudice against or pity for people in that condition. You are opening my eyes and growing me, God. I appreciate it when people open doors for me or allow me to go first—people on a whole are extremely nice to those in less fortunate positions. But still I think that I sense the pity in their eyes or minds. Since when did I become a mind reader? Could it be that I'm projecting onto them my own feelings? Is that why it was such a pleasant surprise to see the many acts of thoughtfulness and kindness that people are still showing nearly 6 months after the stroke?

I seriously doubt that I would still have been as thoughtful except to those closest to me such as Mother. Is this my reward for caring for her, Lord? If so, You have, as usual, given back ten-fold. Thank you Lord, but you know that I did it out of love. You are telling me now that that is exactly what you are looking for. If that is so, then Lee's reward should be immeasurable because he has done so much to make one of your favorite children happy. Help me to always remember and appreciate his acts of love and pass them on. Thanks for Michelle Matthew's advice yesterday about wearing the brace. Most of all, thanks for letting me now show enough vulnerability to let her know that I would be receptive.

Thank you for giving Mother the wisdom to go to the Emergency Room concerning the blister on her leg, which had grown to the size of an egg. Thanks for letting it burst so that it could be treated and please let it be on the way to healing. I trust you Lord not to let any part of Mother need to be amputated and that you will keep her in sound mind and body and reasonably healthy until she comes home to you. Thank you Lord.

And thanks for Rita who cares enough to call and be concerned about both Mother and me. Its daylight now and I am sleepy again so I guess I'll just crawl into this bed in the spare room and nap a little so as not to disturb Lee. He has two weddings to do in the next two days. Thank you for having Jay work with him.

7/7/03

It's 3:30 a.m. and here I am at the keyboard because I can't sleep. It's funny because I was so totally exhausted when I went to bed last night that I remember how that kind of tiredness would have earlier reduced me to tears. What a long way you have brought me. One thing that has me awake is going to bed with numerous small concerns on my mind: having told Michele that Mother and I would attempt to go to the wound center alone to see about Mother's leg because I misunderstood her to say that she could not stay with Mother to speak with the doctor.

There was concern about the work to be put into the Mary Kay Open House that Loretta had proposed for me when I was first attempting to get my business back on track. She and Irie have done most of the work so far and even born most of the expense, duplicating and mailing out my fliers and arranging to come and help.

But as I ponder these things, I realize just how trivial they are compared to the things You have already brought me through. Have I not grown at all? Or have I grown enough to realize when it's time to stop and take stock of my many blessings? I know that if I don't learn my lessons, I am doomed to repeat them and I pray that I have indeed learned them well. There are much larger issues out there and You faithfully see me through them.

I should worry about who will show up at my Open House when you brought people I hadn't seen in years (Vanessa, Shirley, and Sarah) out to pray for me and with me in my time of need? I think not. I just need to remember how you were always there as I sat praying before the window at the hospital with the blizzard swirling outside and could still feel warmth and comfort inside. I knew that You would bring my loved ones safely through the storms and up to the hospital to make sure I knew I was not alone.

Lee came faithfully, even at midnight, when I had chest pains. I did not know at the time that he was also in pain. And Mother and Cat both had aches in their bodies, but still, painfully, walked the long corridors just to visit me.

You even let me make friends of strangers and surrounded me with Your "Angels of Mercy" (Denise, Kathleen, Reba. Donna and Doctor Levitt) to lessen my pain and anxiety any way they could.

Lord, as I entered this room tonight, I remembered coming to it in the wheelchair— having to maneuver it through the doorway and sleep with the door open so that Lee could hear me if I called for help. He would sleep lightly and listen for my every move after having placed everything within easy reach for me. He still listens for my call, to help me up when I fall, but I'm so grateful that I don't need to call nearly as often now. Look where You've brought me from.

So when I go through my everyday concerns about still not being able to control my arm and hand, keep me mindful of the blessings You have bestowed upon me and let me remember: "Don't sweat the small stuff…and it's all small stuff." Now its 4:20 a.m. and I've been up since about 2:30 including bathroom reading time, so I'll get back to bed now and try not to disturb Lee. He has been so good and so patient through all of this. Help me to appreciate and always remember.

7/08/03

I am so blessed. After Lee worked from early this morning until almost dark cleaning out from under the deck, he took the time to put a new screensaver on the computer. Then he called me in to look at it. It is a beautiful scene of a waterfall with soft, soothing music and doves and parrots flying. It also has toy fish swimming and playing just below the water. It was just what I needed to end my day. I don't know why You love me so but I'm so glad You do.

07/09/03

It's 4:45 a.m. I've been tossing and turning since about 4:00. I relaxed before bed with the new screensaver but seemed to have difficulty getting the right arm in a comfortable position. It just troubles me that it wants to stay bent and I picture myself forever with "stroke arm". I will speak to Nicole, the hand therapist, about it even though I'm no longer in therapy, but I fear that she hasn't had enough experience with stroke patients to give me good advice.

Strangely enough, as much as I wish to be physically close to Lee during waking hours, I get almost get irritated when I can't get comfortable and he is right there on my side of the bed. I find myself feeling resentful that he still has not given me a massage or backrub since I had the stroke even though that is the one thing I have longed for most. I have requested it in no uncertain terms and rationalized his not doing it by telling myself that he is afraid to hurt me, but we have been intimate at least twice since that time and he has seen me naked when he helped me in and out of the bathtub, so I don't understand what it is.

I even gave him a one-handed massage

with candlelight and music for our anniversary but he was running a fever that night and I wouldn't expect him to reciprocate. He does so very much for me that I feel guilty wishing for one thing more, and he even took me to the spa to get a massage that the kids gave me as a gift and said that it was the same gift he had planned. He doesn't seem to realize that a massage from his loving hands would feel so much better because then I could moan at will when he put pressure in just the right spot and not feel awkward as with strangers. I guess that I just desire too much from him and he is trying so hard to give me all that I want and need.

I felt that I made progress yesterday. I walked around the patio and yard without feeling the need for the cane. My steps were a little steadier as I focused on the flowers I was walking toward rather than the uneven ground. I walked around the side of the house and even picked fresh mint to make tea. I opened 2 cans of tuna without much difficulty and made sandwiches for Lee and myself. I even sorted and washed 3 loads of laundry, getting them downstairs and up again, and folded one load.

Irie and Loretta modified the flyer I designed for my open house and duplicated, made labels, bought stamps for, and mailed it to my customers. I called as many of them as I could, (about 30) to confirm that they had received the invitation. Michelle has agreed to come over to help with the open house along with Loretta. Everyone is being so nice. Thank you Lord for friends.

Michele is taking Mother to the wound center to see about her leg today. I was going to have Mother pick me up and go with her to speak to the doctor if Michele couldn't stay with her. Mother is concerned that she won't remember some of the things the doctor says. Her memory is getting fuzzy and she might not ask all the necessary questions. She is concerned that her diabetes might cause complications with the leg with disastrous results. I pray not. I will try to remind Michele to press for a home-care nurse to come in and dress the leg twice a day. Right now, Mother has to struggle with it.

Its 5:30 now and I'll try to get a little more sleep in this room before starting my day.

7/10/03

3:30 a.m. – up again, still feeling warm and fuzzy about the successful fellowship that was a result of the loving Mary Kay Customer Appreciation Open House held yesterday. Loretta and Irie really rallied although neither was able to attend the actual event. Loretta's mom had been taken to the emergency room and diagnosed with congestive heart failure (fluid around the heart and lungs) and Irie was called to make a decision on purchasing a home). Still, both checked in to make sure I was ok.

Something unexpected happened with my attitude during preparation. Despite the tiredness I had experienced in gathering items to display, I realized that no matter how few people showed up, its success was not dependent on the money earned. As I looked down into my prayer garden, I determined that we would begin and end our event by truly having God in our midst. My prayer was that everyone who came would leave feeling loved and cared about. And it happened. What a wonderful day!

Thank you God for the new growth within that lets me see the rewards that are richer than money. AMEN

7/14/03

What a blessed day it turned out to be! Rita and I had planned to get together for the day and just hang out, running around wherever our minds took us. Mainly I planned to start the morning in my Prayer Garden and show her how peaceful and beautiful it is with all of the flowers blooming and my little critters running around.

When I awoke to the gray, cloudy skies, however, I was tempted to call it off. Then I figured that God must have something else in mind for us so I started trying to figure out what would make Rita happy. I tried to get a spa appointment for us and, when that fell through, decided to just get together and see how the day would unfold.

As soon as I left it to God, the day fell into place. The sun broke through and I had cantaloupe pieces cut up and ready on the screen porch for Rita and me by the time she arrived with coffee in hand and half a bagel for me. She was transformed the minute she stepped out onto the screen porch. She said that it "smelled like the country" and that it took her back in time to the loving memories of being at her grandmother's farm.

We reminisced together throughout the morning, ending up down on the patio, surrounded by yellow and black finches and numerous other birds of every description that had arrived for breakfast. We spent the entire morning basking in the joy of God's presence and the peaceful serenity of knowing that there was no hurry to go anywhere or do anything except enjoy the glory of a lazy summer day.

We did leave our serenity later to have lake trout and steak fish at Kimmy's and then came back to pick up Mother to go for Italian ice cream at Mikies. We call that our "spoon bouquet" store because on our first visit there, Rita sampled so many flavors, she ended up with a bouquet of tiny spoons in her hand. What a wonderful way to end the day!

It pays to not fret over what appears to be a condition that might change your plans, but to trust that God will work it out to be even better than you had imagined if you will only have faith in him. I'm so glad that we spent that day together.*

I must admit that this had occurred to me

---

* **NOTE:** *One of the things we had discussed was my journals (7/14/03). When I emailed Rita thanking her for the day, she mentioned that my journal entries might be of benefit to others if only I would share them.*

in the past but I dismissed the idea because I thought if I was published before Tina, who had worked so hard on her books and wanted it so badly, Tina would be devastated. This journaling, I know, is not from me. I am convinced that most of it flows from God. Rita asked how I could not share it if it was one of the gifts God gave me. She also said that a true friend would be happy for me if the sharing of my gifts was successful. That was a real eye opener and, as she suggested, it might be time for me to re-evaluate my friendship with Tina if she felt that way.

The name of my book has already come to me. It seems that it should be called "and God said…do the part of it you love to do" quoting from the words he has directed me time and time again to share.

In thinking it over, I guess that I just loved the praise I received from Tina whenever I did something for her; it stroked my ego. It is hard to believe that I let that ego stroking keep me from being obedient to my God. Isn't it funny how we can get caught up? I have decided to just pray on it for now and if I decide to do something about it, Rita said that she has a friend who works at a publishing house whom she would put me in touch with.

7/17/03

I just read a story about a lady who said that she may not have a lot of money but she is doing what she likes and can take the time during the day to enjoy a friend or ponder a passage if she likes. I can truly identify.

Strange as it seems, this will probably go down in my memory as one of the most enjoyable summers that I ever had. I feel free first thing in the morning to make my way out to the patio after breathing in the beauty of the morning and lay out among the flowers and critters to stretch. I look up through the leaves to the patches of blue sky, sometimes even catching a glimpse of one of the larger birds, soaring with wings outstretched. What a sight! Such freedom without a care in the world.

Yesterday, Lee even brought me a breakfast smoothie that he made with fresh banana, wheat germ, and strawberries. It was delicious and energizing. It's so good to be cared for so much and to watch Lee work on the flowers surrounding my prayer garden while he keeps an eye on me. There is no rush for me to finish, to clean up or pursue people in an effort to make more money. We may not have as much liquid cash flow as we have had in the past but we can go on vacation when we want and can still afford to have date night every week. This is truly a blessing. Most important of all, we are taking the time to enjoy each other. What a blessing! Thank you, Lord.

I could even take the time to really enjoy going with Michele and the boys to watch Cameron's tennis lesson this morning. Michele and I sat in canvas chairs in the shade of a tree while Ethan played with a friend nearby. Then we went to pick up lunch to take back to Michele's and Everett joined us, emerging from his office downstairs. Michele showed me her beautiful flowers in her yard before returning me home for a nap. What a wonderful life. God is truly blessing me and mine and I will be forever grateful.

7/18/03 - GUILT

I'm up by 5 this morning, partly because of the hip discomfort but mostly because of guilt. Last night Mother called to say that she believed that the shunt in her arm was clogged. She couldn't feel the pulse beat that is usually distinct. She debated going to the hospital but I suggested that she wait until this morning when she would be at dialysis and they could let her know for sure. When she said that there would be no way for her to get to the hospital from dialysis if she needed to have it unclogged, I suggested that she take money enough for a cab. I never even asked Lee if he would mind our picking her up and taking her to the hospital where she wouldn't be alone for the painful procedure.

Lee has been working really hard to

complete 3 videotapes that have been requested by this weekend and I felt guilty asking him to stop his work. I'm afraid that I am getting callous when it comes to Mother, partly because I see now that others willingly take on some of the responsibility of caring for her and partly because I don't feel that I'm any real help when I just go along for the ride and am unable to make any real contribution. Mother seems to feel better if I am there but I think it is just a matter of habit. No matter what the reason, if my presence is a comfort to her, I should try to be there for her whenever I can.

Earlier in the week, she mentioned that her Para-transit tickets were running out. I was willing to ride down with her to get them but unwilling to walk the distance required to actually go in and make the purchase. I walk alone further than that every Friday night when we go to the movies and Lee drops me off before parking the car.

I know how it feels just to have the reassurance that someone is there for you so I don't understand my own behavior. I will check with Lee this morning about picking her up if necessary and will call to let her know. It is only 15 minutes away but I'm reluctant to add another thing to his already-full plate. Help me Lord to be of help without overburdening others. AMEN

7/28/03- INTIMACY

It is 4:20 a.m. and I have been tossing and turning for about 2 hours. I finally decided to get up even though I am still sleepy. I was so sleepy when I went to bed last night but the thoughts were nagging at me that I wasn't showing any intimacy toward Lee even though I desire him a lot. I just don't know how to show him, especially since I still can't even get my right arm and leg to move properly to wrap around him.

It was not only since the stroke, however, that I felt inadequate when it comes to showing him how much I desire him. I'm really not sure what to do about it. He is so patient with me but doesn't like to discuss things so my attempts to resolve things of this nature have failed in the past. Meanwhile, when he gets to the breaking point, we are physically intimate but don't make love the way we used to (no kissing and I can't remember when or if he has ever looked into my eyes).

I still know how blessed I am to have him show how much he cares in so many other ways; surrounding me with flowers he grows, watching over me as I exercise outside to be sure I don't hurt myself, etc., but I don't know how to give back. This is probably a dilemma that will plague me for the next 38 years of our marriage. Meanwhile, I'll continue to be grateful that God gave him to me to love.

I am getting more concerned about my right arm, fingers, leg, and foot. The fingers have definitely curved to the left; the arm wants to draw up and won't lie out flat if I lay on my stomach. The leg is getting stronger but the foot still won't bend back on its own, and the toes are curling under and to the right. I'm going to see the outpatient doctor at Kernan on Wednesday for my periodic checkup and will mention these things to him, but he didn't seem really concerned or helpful the first time I saw him.

I am searching out support groups in the area and have seen an article in the stroke magazine about a device (*SAEBO FLEX*) that might aid in regaining movement in my arm. I have managed through exercise to get it to the point where I can make it lift, with control, when I lay flat on my back so I guess that's progress.

All these things on my mind along with my looking into details of our anticipated trip to Disneyworld in December are probably the reason I can't sleep. I know that I will take a long nap during the day and I just thank God for the freedom to do that. I will try to take it as soon as I need it and not put it off until it throws off my schedule for sleep at night.

Well, I'm sleepy now, so I guess I'll crawl into this bed in the spare room so as not to disturb Lee.

7/29/03

A repeat performance of last night—awake for about two hours. It's about 4:32 a.m. I kept trying to keep my arm straight but awoke to it bent up to my face. I have visions of it staying that way and it scares me. I am going to investigate the apparatus that I saw in the stroke magazine that is supposed to enable you to use the weak arm and hand affectively again. I'm almost sure that insurance won't cover it but I'll find a way to pay for it. Tomorrow, I'll inquire about the advisability of it when I return to Kernan for a checkup.

I find myself wondering if I should have chosen the tPA option that might have broken up the clot in my brain right after the stroke. Statistics say that there is a 6% chance that it might cause bleeding in the brain which causes the patient to die. That means that there is a 94% chance that it won't, but 6% seemed like a big chance when it was my life on the line.

Should I have had the faith that God

would not take me if it was not my time to go? Somehow I'm convinced that God needed me to go through this whole experience, with North Arundel Hospital, Kernan, and Lee this summer, to prepare me for something. So I pray that I can accept whatever I am going through with the knowledge that it will come out ok in the end.

This morning, Lee and I are taking Mother to Bayview hospital to see a doctor about the pocket on her esophagus that the doctor at North Arundel Hospital found. I pray that it is something that can be removed successfully without any permanent damage.

Well, I'm going to sleep a little now to gain strength for the day. Help me in my weakness, Lord, to have faith in all You do and know that it is for my good. I'm always saying that I'm one of Your favorite people. I don't know how I know that but I'm convinced that whatever You allow will be for my ultimate good. Thank you Father.

7/31/03

I had deep concerns about Mother and my lack of ability to see to her sense of well being without endangering my own health. I had even told her that she would pretty much be on her own going to appointments unless there was something happening there that required me to hear it. That sounded very callous but I was afraid that I was falling back into the old pattern which would lead to overwork and stress trying to do everything myself. And now, I was even involving Lee because I have not yet been recertified to drive.

I also think that part of my attitude was the result of feeling like my going with Mother was more of a hindrance than a help, having to be pushed or trying to slowly walk to wherever our assigned appointment was. I had also tried to convince Mother of the wisdom of moving into a Senior Citizen building where, for a fee, they prepared meals, cleaned up, and assisted with baths and medicines. What I failed to consider was one of the most important things You taught me through this stroke experience -- that independence lets one maintain dignity and self-esteem. We have come full circle now, where you are tying it all together for me.

The courses in self-esteem that you encouraged me to teach, the feeling of the loss of dignity at times in the hospital, etc., all come together so that I can handle this situation with love. Thank you Father. I will follow your lead and invite Cat, Byron, Michele, and Mike to team up with me to make Mother's days remaining on earth as full of joy and dignity as we are able.

I will list the things provided by the Senior Citizen apartments and get suggestions on ways we can most easily provide them while she stays in her present apartment. I know that people, especially seniors, don't like to be uprooted. The advantage is that she already lives in a handicap-equipped apartment so that alleviates some safety concerns.

The fact that Byron also stays there helps

with the concern of having someone to check on her almost daily and to pick up extraneous items, as needed. She also has Rodney, the maintenance man and Kenny, the dialysis bus driver looking out for her. She must be pleasing in your sight to have so many people looking out for her when she is unable to fend for herself.

I will strongly suggest that she give up driving because she has told me that she feels she is going blind. I pray that you don't let that happen but that it is your way of encouraging her to stop driving before some of her other health problems might cause her to hurt herself or others. I will suggest that she take a cab to her appointment this morning and in the future, I will arrange a ride through the Department of Aging to get her there. She can take a cab back and not have to wait. These are some of the other suggestions You have given me this morning:

Bathing—she has a bar in the shower and a shower chair. I can investigate the other bathtub safety features mentioned in the stroke magazine.

Eating—she has located her crock pot that can cook while she is out, softening food until it is easily chewable. Eating at the Senior place is not as desirable to her because she does not always want to dress in more than a duster for meals and they may not prepare foods she likes to eat. We can shop together every 1-2 weeks, riding the carts, and that will also help Lee with groceries. He can take us in the time he might have had to shop. We can even have lunch at the mall. Mother can be given a pad and encouraged to jot down items as she thinks of them or runs out. Any special dishes or leftovers we might want to share can be brought to her house once per week or whenever we accompany her to an appointment. We should call first to find out if there is anything she needs picked up while we are on our way.

Dr appointments – we should take turns, taking and bring her on the days and times that we decide ahead of time most conveniently fit into everyone's schedule. These schedules are flexible and the appointments will be scheduled, as nearly as possible, around the planned times (Tuesday and Thursday – non-dialysis days). Mother will be encouraged to jot down symptoms of discomforts (or I will maintain a list) and they will be sent to the doctor If no one can stay to see the doctor during her appointment, permission will be asked ahead of time for the doctor to give a time we can call him for results or recommendations. Michele or I will call.

Medications—NeighborCare will deliver prescriptions to dialysis.

Wheelchair—paperwork will be picked up from doctor Ng and sent/delivered to health and mobility. Mother's furniture will be rearranged (Mike/Byron) to accommodate.

8/10/03

Wayne is coming! He's bringing Judy, Erica, Marc, Tammi (Marc's wife), and Marc's son,

Brandon. B.J. couldn't make the trip because he and his wife, Ami, just gave birth to their first child, Brianna, on August 1 (Mike and Heather's birthday). We are so excited about seeing them and I can't believe how much I was stressing yesterday morning over what had to be done to prepare a simple cookout for them in the backyard.

Lee had volunteered to do the work, but I was stressing over the food, the number of people, etc. Thank you, Lord, for getting me grounded again by Lee and Michele telling me that they are handling it and, most of all, by Your calling my attention to all the beautiful gifts with which You had surrounded me. Had I even had noticed them? You sent young squirrels to amuse me with their antics, yellow finches and a Blue Jay to show me beauty with their colors, and even caused 3 new flowers to bloom on my favorite vine which Lee had nurtured from last summer. Forgive me Lord for not acknowledging all that You so generously give.

I began today differently, thanking You for

the safe trip I know You'll allow Wayne's family to make. I pray that I remember to focus always on what will make them enjoy their visit most instead of how my house looks.

Please bless the meeting planned for Wednesday to divide the duties of taking care of Mother's needs so that we can take some of the stress away from her. She is still driving but has periods where she doesn't see so well and always feels better if someone else accompanies her to the doctor. My contribution to the team is to coordinate the effort, making sure all players are in place and equipped with all necessary information. I will also act as a database for all test results so that everyone knows where to go to get the information.

I have relieved her of the burden of bill paying by putting it all online. I pray that I can be of most help this way without adding to Lee's burden by having him pick up and take us places in my attempt to do my part. Thank you, Lord. You are showing me how I can use the knowledge you have equipped me with right here in the family without ever leaving home. It is again coming together. You are awesome.

8/13/03

Thank you, Father, for the wonderful memories you have allowed us to build over the past few days. The cookout was great with everyone talking and laughing and taking pictures. I can't wait to put them together in a memory book. There was more than enough food with Lee working diligently on homemade potato salad, hot dogs, burgers, and shopping for pie, cookies, and chips.

He worked from early morning, stringing lights across the patio and cleaning the yard and screen porch. Michele prepared pasta/seafood salad, stuffed mushrooms and arrived early to help finish preparations. About 23 people came with even Robert bringing his friend, Robin, and her daughter, and Byron bringing his friend, Rose, and her son.

With Wayne and the gang here, crabs

were scarfed up and Wayne even cleaned and picked a couple for me. Everyone truly enjoyed themselves and I thank you Father. The last folks didn't leave until about 10:30 p.m. and we all slept the most pain-free, trouble-free sleep we had slept in ages. That is how I knew for sure that your hand was on this place.

We loved Marc's wife Tammi, and she and Michele really bonded as did Cameron and Marc's son, Brandon. Wayne seems to have settled in, no longer trying to be boisterous and Judi seems truly happy. They came with good news and pictures of B.J.'s new baby, Brianna.

Cliff couldn't be here because he is going through an illness that even puzzles the doctors with swelling and no feeling in the bottoms of his feet. Please help him get well, Lord, and help Cat to be able to bear up under whatever is to come. (August 2003)

We rented wheelchairs for Mother and me and took Wayne's gang down to the Science Center yesterday to see Titanic footage at the Imax. We thoroughly enjoyed ourselves but were a little disappointed that we missed the show at the planetarium. The good news, though, was that we were given all our admission money back as well as 6 free passes to come again because of a broken wheelchair lift. We later bought chicken and enjoyed each other at Mother's house. I again had a blessed night's sleep. Thank you Lord.

Wayne and crew moved on to continue their vacation today, heading to Virginia to see Judi's sister before going back to Ohio to visit Judi's parents and then to see B.J., Ami, and Brianna before returning home. Thank you for traveling mercies, Lord, and blessed memories.

AMEN

8/21/03 - Progress

Praise Jehovah, Lord God Almighty; praise Jehovah, Everlasting King; we praise Your name!!! This morning, when I awoke, I was able to move my right thumb, pointer, and little fingers, almost at will. Yesterday, I could move my right arm without first lifting my shoulder. Healing is taking place! Thank you, Lord.

While outside this morning, I walked, unaided by cane, completely around the house and down the right-of-way the entire length of my neighbor, Anna's, yard! What a feeling of independence! I kept wiggling my fingers all day like a baby who just discovered she has hands. The first thing I did after waking from my nap was to test to see that they still worked. I couldn't wait to show Lee what I could do, and he was his usual crazy self. He stuck one finger up his nose and said, "but can you do this?" ☺ There will always be humor with him around.

I called Michele, Mike, Rita, Michelle, and Cat to share the good news. Mother had concerns of her own so I did not get into this with her. By nighttime, I found that I could also make my wrist flop forward at will. It was a great day! It was hard to wipe the smile off my face.

8/22/03

I've been awake since about 4:00 thinking about Mother's situation with her growing inability to find the right words to finish her sentences. It seems a lot like the aphasia that I saw while I was at Kernan. Could that be another reason that You had me go through this experience? I know that this frustrates and probably frightens her as she wonders if she is losing her memory. Please help me, Lord, to find someone who can help her so she will have peace of mind knowing that she is not alone. That means so much. I will try to reach Doctor Pieri today to get a recommendation of another doctor. Meanwhile, please give me words of comfort that will help. AMEN

9/1/03

I had to write before going to bed because I knew that if I did not get it off my mind, I would not sleep well. Tonight I cried again out of helplessness. I am trying to do everything I can for Mother without involving Lee as much as possible, but he keeps being dragged into it anyway. He is already trying to provide all my needs and most of my wants but yesterday, when I tried to help Mother lay out her medication over the phone, she knocked the pills over 3 times.

She takes 11 kinds of medicine in the mornings and 9 at night and a lot of them look alike. Her eyesight is failing and she is doing the best she can to stay out of a nursing home.

Lord, please help me to help her win this battle. Lee took me up there this evening to help her and we missed going to a movie because there was so much medication to sort out. He ate by himself while he was out because he had not eaten much today and I just had peanut butter and jelly when we got home.

He was rather silent with me because I know he is concerned that I'm again taking on too much. Michele and Mike were supposed to take and bring Mother to and from her eye appointment tomorrow but Michele is sick and Mike has a meeting. Mother will most likely get drops in her eyes but will still have to take a cab in both directions. She will have to do the same on Thursday when she goes to the hospital for the removal of the temporary catheter.

I'm trying to save Lee to take us to meet the Geriatric specialist next week. I really need to connect with a Senior Caregiver Support group so that I can get some idea as to how to handle this. Please, Lord, give me strength of mind and body to do what is necessary and realize when I have to give this over to you. I already know that I cannot do it without you. I pray the serenity prayer and pray that you will not let Mother feel that she has been deserted. And please, Lord, let Lee know how much I love him for caring so much. AMEN

9/11/03

Awake since 3:30 for no particular reason. No aches or pains, thank goodness. I was sitting in the screen house yesterday just thanking God for the wonder of another pain-free day and the ability and freedom to do whatever I had the urge to attempt. That morning, I decided to walk out and check the progress of my tomatoes on my giant 12-15 foot tomato plants and then just stood looking up at the beauty of the blue skies on a humidity-free morning.

When the urge struck me to check out the condition of the inside of the camper, I found that mice or chipmunks had left their calling cards in every drawer, so I decided to take hose, bucket and cleaner and restore freshness. I unzipped the windows and thoroughly enjoyed wiping down everything as the sunshine and fresh breezes blew in. When I finally finished, about 2 hours later, I had a great sense of accomplishment and went to lie out on my lounge in the screen house, just contemplating savoring the giant tomato sandwich from my bush. Lee cut it for me along with some turkey and it was delicious! Then I lay back, guilt-free and took a nap in the screen house, undisturbed by phones or guilt over unmade beds. What a life! I shall always remember this summer.

Tonight, I will get to go to my first Stroke Survivors meeting. I am so excited!

9/17/03

For some reason, I was unable to sleep tonight (or I guess it was last night since it is 2:30 a.m.) I have dreamed of someone who is already dead for two nights in a row. Night before last, it was Daddy, and last night, it was

Uncle Ernest, but they both were very much alive in my dreams. I was really very tired on both nights so I find it hard to imagine why I didn't sleep soundly.

A hurricane is predicted to strike on Thursday night and Lee and I spent the morning preparing by taking down the screen house and camper and pulling in the lawn furniture and hibiscus plants. Mother spent a contented day with anticipation of her new helper who comes to do some light housekeeping and helps with her bath. It seems that things might finally be coming together for her with people at the Department of Aging taking up her fight with the transportation people at MTA.

I was able to find some decent fares online for our flight to Disney and I booked them tonight. For some reason, I had the urge to call Mike yesterday evening to be sure that everything was all right. It was, and we just chatted briefly about the hurricane and hung up. I pray that this uneasy feeling is unfounded and I'll just trust the Lord to keep me and my loved ones safe. I usually wish for time to make a journal entry without being sleepy but now that I have the time, I have run out of things to say. I'll go back to bed soon.

Lee doesn't seem to be coughing tonight, although his cough during the day concerns me. I am wearing the shirt that says "God, grant me the serenity to accept the things I cannot change, the courage to change the things that I can, and the wisdom to know the difference." That is my prayer.

I was reading Oprah's "Things I Know For Sure" where she talked about being able to make a difference, and it struck me how my attitude has changed from trying to make a difference in someone else's life to trying to make a difference in my own. I rationalized this by saying that if I made a difference for me, God would be pleased because I would have helped one of his favorite people. Maybe that's a bit arrogant of me but I truly believe that I am one of his favorites, though sometimes I don't act like I believe it. Like now, I keep waiting to hear the footsteps of someone coming to do me harm when I profess to believe that God would not let anything bad happen to me.

Why am I so confused? I will just pray Jebez's prayer, that God will keep his hand upon us and let no harm come to us; believe, and then go contentedly to sleep knowing that God has it all in control.

When did I stop speaking directly to you in my journal, Father, and start dictating a narrative? When did I get too distracted to spend time in Your word in the morning? It seems that I just got too caught up in the beauty of your natural gifts; the birds, the flowers, the trees, to want to miss any of it looking down in a book. But is that so wrong? I think not, now that I've written it. You would not have surrounded me with such beauty and filled me with such joy when I behold it if it would displease You when I did so. Thank you for the gifts and the ability to enjoy them. My eyes are getting heavy now so I'll go contentedly to sleep knowing that you have it all in control.

Thank you Father. AMEN

9/17/03

I finally sent a letter to Denise Harding's supervisor with a copy to Denise, telling her how grateful I was for the help and comfort she gave at the onset of my stroke. I'm really glad that I got that done.

9/18/03

They say that a devastating hurricane—Isabel—may be on the way. Everyone is taking precautions because it has the potential to be the worse one since 1933. The Federal government is closing its offices at noon and the schools in the area are all closed for the day. We have put down the screen house and camper, and brought in the lawn chairs. One thing that I have learned from this stroke is not to regret the things that I didn't do yesterday but, instead, to do the things today that may make things better.

I was about to feel guilty about not inviting Mother down to ride out the storm with us but told her which room to run to in case the storm hit. Instead of regretting that decision, I called to tell her to bring a packed overnight bag with her when the senior bus picked her up for her 2 doctor's appointments this morning and have the bus drop her off here. That way, she won't be alone should the storm hit. I also remembered to have the courtesy to check with Lee before calling her. You are truly making me more thoughtful.

I awoke this morning thinking of the items I should add to our stash in the little cubby in the laundry room with just enough space for the 3 of us to squeeze in should it become necessary. I have already equipped it with blankets, pillows, plastic, water, flashlight, and peanut butter. I was blessed to find a little battery-operated radio up here on the desk as well as a push-on light. I included Band-Aids, tape, ointment, paper towels, scissors, dried fruit, packaged candy, depends, and cell phones on the list.

I'm sleepy again so I guess I'll rest awhile and then pack those in. Whatever the storm does, I know that you will protect my loved ones and me and I thank you Lord. AMEN

9/30/03- How Blessed I Am!!!

I woke up this morning with a grin on my face that is hard to erase. When I opened my eyes and saw the beautiful, sunny, blue-skied day, that even added more joy. I realized that I was completely on Lee's side of the bed (I don't know how he slept in the little space I had left for him), and that my side was almost undisturbed. When the weather gets cooler, I have the tendency to seek the warmth of his body while I sleep.

I rolled over and over back to my side of the bed with complete abandon. I guess that I was still feeling the joy of my dream last night where I was running around with Michele trying on all kinds of crazy clothes in a dressing room and feeling carefree. At one point, we saw a bow-legged guy when we were outside and he was unattractive, but later I thought what it would be like to be loved and adored, making love without restrictions, looking adoringly at each other again.

I felt guilty for a moment until I realized that God already gave me that gift in Lee. He keeps that special feeling alive, taking me to Bed and Breakfast places where we can awake in each other's arms after sleeping spoon-style, wrapped around each other's bodies; he doesn't feel inhibited from making love on a blanket in front of a roaring fire or in a Jacuzzi outside our bedroom.

He still has that caring side that allows him to work in the yard just close enough to watch over me when I'm having one of my "dare-devil" days, trying new things while walking with or without my cane; and Lee even remembers to pick up fresh fruit and smoothie makins' when I have expressed the desire to start my day with one. Oh, how very blessed I am!!!

There is no need to fantasize or ever stray. You have given it all to me in Lee. Thank you,

Lord.

10/03/03

I met a new friend and Stroke survivor, Irma Simon and husband, Rogers. I felt a spirit-to-spirit connection right away. I can see Jesus joy just radiating from her face.

10/05/03

I woke up at about 4 this morning but just lay there content, nestled in the tuck of Lee's warm body snuggled around me, thinking of ways to help solve Mother's eating dilemma and coming up with ideas. I later got up and put them on the computer. Things seem to be turning around for her now that she has a helper, Barbara, coming in 5 times each week for a couple of hours. Michele and I think that part of Mother's "down" attitude was caused by loneliness. Mother's blood pressure is still not under control. Friday, they almost put her in the hospital again when it shot up to 260 but they managed to get it down to 200 so they agreed to let her go home.

Lee and I accomplished a lot around here yesterday and I thank you, God, for giving me the strength and determination to keep at it. I did take a break for a nap, though, before I got too tired. Lee tackled the basement and later we took a break to have dinner and TV time together before he went back to do more and I tackled bills. It was a good and fruitful day.

10/06/03

I went to the Emergency Room with persistent pain in my left side. They diagnosed it as *gallstones* and recommended surgery. I opted to wait until I see my new doctor to see what she recommends. I'm not happy.

10/09/03

Hallelujah! Thank you, Jesus! The final piece of documentation arrived that was needed for Mother's package to get her accepted into her new apartment. She needed the proof of income from Social Security and after 2 failed mailings, they promised to fax it to me but said that could only be done after 4 p.m. I left the fax on for four hours and nothing came. But this morning, Lee told me that a fax was trying to get through. I turned the machine on and, lo and behold, there it came, at 9 in the morning. Look at God working! And just in time so that the leasing manager could approve the application and we could get the letter off to Mother's apartment complex to get her out of her lease 30 days prior to moving.

Martina came over for some Mary Kay product tonight and we praised God together. Had she not warned me about getting assets out of Mother's name nearly a year ago, a lot of help that we received recently wouldn't have been possible. What an awesome God You are! And I will pass knowledge on to others who might also be helped by it.

It was a good day, concluding with seeing my new-found Christian sister, Irma, who is also a stroke survivor. She responded to my invitation to join us at the Stroke Survivors meeting and had also called to participate in the Pepper study. I guess I'm already passing on knowledge and just hadn't realized how much. Somehow, when we do things that would please You, it doesn't take a lot of forethought. It just naturally flows out of us. Thank you, Lord. May I continue to be a blessing.

I went to see the new doctor, Lisa Goldberg, recommended by Neal's mom, and I really like her. She changed some of my medication and gave me samples. Best of all, she truly listened to what I had to say. Thank you for a replacement for Doctor Pieri. I pray that Mother will be just as pleased when she meets with her new doctor.

My head is swimming with ideas to help with Mother's move. One special thing I want to do for her is to take a piece of the huge rhododendron bush that she planted outside of her apartment and loves so much, and root a piece of it in a pretty pot to go to her new home. How happy that will make her to bring a little bit of the life she had at the last home she and Daddy shared. I feel You smiling at that idea and I'm so glad it pleases You.

I've been awake since about 4 a.m., partly because of all of these ideas and partly, I fear, because of the onions I ate about 8 o'clock on the sub that Lee bought for us to share. I may be sleepy later but I've learned not to lie there tossing and turning but to "do the part of it I love to do". It's funny how often those words of wisdom keep popping up. I will definitely share those words with the world even if little of the other of my ponderings is put out for the world to see.

It's funny now...I thought I felt a feeling of sadness from You when I said that. I would never want to disappoint You. I guess that it is just the fear of leaving another work half finished like I did the "AnnieBand" that keeps me from attempting one more thing. But, when I think of it, maybe my portion of the task was to get the idea out there, and then, like a relay runner, pass the baton on to the next runner. Help me to run my portion of the race to the best of my ability, Lord, and never let me fail to take up a new torch to begin another. Perhaps that is why you gave me this visionary spirit… to jumpstart others on this race called life. Use me Lord.

10/13/03

I'm getting stronger and more adventurous! This morning was beautiful. When I looked out and saw a lady taking a walk, I had the urge to do the same. I got to the corner by the Marino's house and just kept walking! I walked all the way around Scotts Glen, grinning up at the beautiful Fall sky and crunching through dried leaves. Oh, the freedom I felt! Thank you, Lord.

10/14/03

Sometimes events can be mixed blessings. Clients started calling and placing orders which was a good thing, but a couple also wanted to come over to see some things. I would normally welcome this promise of extra income, but as I started to try to get orders ready for mailing, folding priority mailboxes with one hand, standing unsteadily on my feet, I started dropping things (like my draw full of samples, on the floor where its contents joined the styrofoam peanuts I had spilled earlier.

While dodging that mess and trying to tape the top and bottom of the box I was sending, I felt frustration really beginning to build up. Top that off with the fact that I had to successfully step over the mess to get to the computer to type out labels and a copy of the orders I was sending out, and I was an emotional mess! I finally got it done, and sent the packages off with Lee while still thinking of the lady (Neal's mom) who was coming over at 3:30 to get a glamour makeover.

I decided to give Michelle (my Mary Kay team member) a quick call for help, but when I started to talk to her, my voice cracked after I had told her that I needed her at 3:30. Trying to hold back the tears, I just said I'd call her back. When I pulled myself together, I called her back and didn't have to say more than a few words before she said, "Say no more, I'll be there." Thank you, God, for understanding friends. She came and we three had a wonderful time together. Michele and I made plans to do other work together, and when I noted that her MS had left her weak on one side and I was weak on the other, she replied, "Together, we can stand tall".

10/15/03

Today I began a new phase in my life. I went down to begin evaluation for acceptance into the Pepper study being done by the VA hospital at the University Hospital. If I am accepted, I will receive free therapy on my weak arm and leg while they do studies to see how my brain responds. I am excited and confident that I will be accepted if it is the right thing for me. God is on my side.

10/19/03

Hallelujah! Thank you Jesus! Another breakthrough! This morning while lying on my back, I was able to bring my weak arm all the way up past my shoulder and back down *with control!* Then, I could lift it from elbow to hand, up and away from my body (elbow still rested on the bed). What a breakthrough! I feel God reconnecting my body and it is truly wonderful. When I think of the trivial concerns I had about my body before (scar from surgery, varicose veins, etc.), I now see how unimportant those things really are. Thank you, Jesus.

I went for a walk because it was such a beautiful Fall day. I walked all the way up to Perthshire Path and stood at the fence of the yard with the pond. There is such peace back there. I'm sure God is there as I listen to the soft sound of water tumbling over the rocks and into the pond. I have to smile as I look at the faces of the gnome statues that stand and lie at either end of the footbridge. I wonder if the homeowner there knows what joy his handiwork brings to others as they pass. I'm tempted to knock on his door and tell him but decided against it. His house sits right at the edge of the woods but I reassure myself that there is nothing to fear there because God is watching over me. That is the furthest I have walked since the stroke and my next goal is to walk all the way to Gwen's house.

When I came back, I walked around back and picked what is probably the last tomato I'll get from the bushes this season. I pulled one of the chairs over and really enjoyed watching the wind cause the leaves to come swirling down. I just sat there for awhile, looking up and smiling. I was feeling content and remembering such a time when I was about 10 or 11, sitting out in Daddy's rowboat in the backyard of our house in Turner Station. I didn't really know God at that time. I only knew that I felt safe and at peace with the big, colorful leaves surrounding me. Little did that little girl know that God already had plans of how He would use her to spread joy though the world. I'm sure that I don't have a complete picture even now, but I'm glad that I have gotten to know Him much better now.

10/20/03

Thank you God, for the birth of M&M, the name Michelle and I gave to our joint Mary Kay mission. Bless us Lord as we work together to fulfill the works that will grow out of it; doing the parts of it we love to do while enriching our lives and others' and enjoying the journey along the way. It feels so right that I just know it is from You. Speak through us as we put our plans in place with each of us thinking of the other first. Thank you, Lord.

10/25/03

I have just finished reading a part of this journal and have really enjoyed it. It just might make good reading for others in the future. I am excited about our upcoming plans to go to

Rita's for Thanksgiving and stay for 2 nights at a nice hotel to celebrate Lee's birthday. Help me to make it enjoyable for him, Lord, please. He has done so much to brighten my days.

Thank you for helping me finalize the details of Mother's upcoming move to the brand new Senior Apartments at Parkview. Help her to be happy and content as she settles in there. Thank you, Lord.

10/28/03

It is so good to know that I've got God on my side when temptation rears its ugly head. We had started M&M, a partnership I know was inspired by God, and He had given me the outline of how it should go. It made perfect unselfish sense until money was actually added into the equation. Then greed took over my logic temporarily. It didn't even require much money but Satan will get you as cheaply as he can just to bring you down and make you feel that much more ashamed of your fall.

But God was standing by and He let me

put up a struggle all day as I wrestled with this problem. It all happened when it was time to divide the money Michelle and I had earned during our first week of partnership. God's plan was that we would take turns putting in orders from M&M's funds, thereby giving both of us Seminar credits. Michelle would get the first order. But I was keeping the records and had inadvertently deposited one of M&M's checks with mine. When I saw that the amount earned when added to mine would give me enough credit to earn the next highest commission, it made sense to me to maximize the profit by changing God's plan.

Of course, I would also have to chase down three other consultants to get them to order. I had also, as part of the God-inspired plan, decided that we should open a new bank account together with Michelle's name as the primary because I already had an account at that bank in my name. But Satan told me that I already had an account we could use that was lying dormant and that I would be giving away *my power* if I did it the way it was originally planned. What power??

Whatever power I have comes from the Lord and you have no idea how physically hard it is to write this now; my head feels tight and there is tightness in my back. I even heard a loud noise outside trying to distract me but I will write it anyhow.

This morning I will call Michelle and we will pray together. Then I will invite her to go with me to the bank and together we will open the account of our God-based business. I will tell her of yesterday's struggles and thank her for being so connected with God that she never fought against me in any of the decisions I made yesterday, no matter how little sense they made. God was showing me that she could be trusted to do the things that made sense for this partnership. Thank You God.

The tightness is easing up now. "*Resist the Devil and he shall flee*." I know that I can't do it alone and I thank You God that You never leave me or forsake me.

10/31/03—Camping

We decided to take Cameron and Ethan camping. It was Ethan's first time, and what a time we had! Ethan became Granddaddy (Lee's) "shadow", doing everything from helping him fry hotdogs to helping him "fix" the camper. We let both kids take part in the Halloween costume parade and Cameron won one of the 10 prizes for best costume, dressed as "Cameron Potter", and equipped with his new Harry Potter glasses he had to start wearing this year.

We had a ball, roasting marshmallows on the end of sticks Lee whittled for us. Ethan ate more "clean" ones right out of the bag than we ate of those we roasted. The boys and Lee took a ride in a paddleboat and fed doughnuts to the geese while I took pictures from the shore. Lee couldn't figure out why it was so hard to paddle until he found that Cameron had stuck his feet between the paddle and the boat.

We wrapped up our trip by collecting beautiful golden yellow leaves that were falling from a big tree (some hadn't even fallen yet and Cameron climbed up on a picnic table to help them along). Cameron had a ball in the game room with $5.00 worth of quarters from his prize money and Ethan got to drive on a road in the campground while sitting next to his Granddaddy, So, in spite of 4 falls for Ethan and 2 for me, we made a wonderful memory. The near 80-degree weather was a blessed gift as well. Thank you Lord.

11/03/03

The Doctor has told me that I should have surgery to remove my gallbladder because of the gallstones. She said it should only take a week to recuperate and I hope she is right. I want to wait and get a second opinion since the people at the hospital who first diagnosed them have not sent her the report or the films yet, but it is getting so close to the holidays that I hate to think of spoiling them with surgery.

Our plans include Thanksgiving at Rita's, Lee's birthday celebration at the special hotel, Christmas, and the Disney trip. Then in January, Lee has scheduled surgery for his foot. But I will not worry about things over which I have no control. You have brought us safely through this year, dealing with something that was life changing, and I have faith that You will also bring us through this next step, wiser and loving each other.

Mother's move is scheduled for less than 2 weeks from now and people are already helping her to get ready. I thank you for granting this gift and for giving me the beauty of yesterday when I again collected colorful leaves in the backyard in preparation for the *WELCOME* display I will make for Mother's new apartment.

Thank you Lord for the things Lee and I are accomplishing to make our home even more warm and loving (Lee just made an arrangement of pots of African Violets on the table under my office window after I cleaned it off. Life is good and I don't know why I stress over what may happen tomorrow when I know that You will turn it into good. Thank you Lord. AMEN

11/5/03

It is just shortly after 6 a.m. and I have been awake for more than an hour, lying in bed and pondering the things Michele said to me yesterday. How true they were—that I have fallen back into the same pattern that I was in prior to the stroke—trying to do everything for Mother and feeling guilty about those I can't do. How strange that is since I'm always quoting the prayer "God, grant me the serenity to accept the things I cannot change, the courage to change the things I can, and the wisdom to know the difference." Thank you for sending me a reminder through Michele that, if we don't learn from what we go through, we are destined to repeat it.

Yesterday, I found myself stressed over finding a way to get Mother to an appointment and resenting Lee for showing intolerance when I had him pick her up and take both of us to get it done. I even tried to push her wheelchair, though barely able to balance myself getting in and out of the elevator. He had already gone to get blood work done that morning and I don't know what health issues he is going through.

I have fallen into the guilt pattern that I thought I gave up when I cut Tina loose; only this time, I'm allowing Mother to put me in that place. When I spoke about my upcoming gallstone surgery and mentioned that the Internet report said that the condition, if left untreated, could be fatal, Mother asked, "Isn't that the week I'm supposed to move?" I know she loves me but sometimes human nature lets a person focus on his or her own needs first, so I'd better start acting human.

Without having to announce my change in priorities, I have decided to devote one hour per day to Mother's needs, sticking to my original resolution to do my part from the computer and phone. I will do these things after naptime in the afternoon, so as not to get caught up in them in the morning and have them spill over into the rest of the day. I feel that a lot of Lee's resentment comes from the fact that he is trying to look out for my health and my needs and then he sees me let Mother do things which will be detrimental.

I say how important he is to me but have again not shown it. I have resolved to dedicate at least an hour each day to doing something just for him. I know that he doesn't expect much and, God forgive me, I haven't given much. Please help me to take the time and open my heart and mind to see and do the things that would make his life more pleasant. He doesn't require that I put a lot of work in the house and is always happier giving than receiving, but everyone has human wants and needs and he has inferred in the past that, if I really loved him, I'd know things that pleased him. You have not spoken the words out loud, yet I know what pleases You, so I pray that You'll help me see his needs as well.

One more thing that I resolve to do is to get back to exercising to work the muscles You have restored. Somehow, I had put that on hold, waiting for the Pepper Study to bring it back. Thanks for these revelations, Lord. And please bless me that I may be a blessing.

Would you, also, please watch over Mike with whatever condition is causing his chest pains, watch over Mother in whatever is causing her back pain, and bless Michele as she watches out for and helps us all. Most of all, please bless Lee, and again, I thank you for making him my life partner. He is a proof, greater than any other on earth, of how much You truly love me. AMEN

11/6/03

Isn't it fun to be spontaneous? Lee suggested that we ride back up to the campground together to pay the man for repairing the camper and see about the cost of storage. I was ready in less than half an hour. We had some scary time on the way when a storm rolled in spawning a tornado and the storm was moving our way. I wanted to pull over into a building until the storm had passed but Lee insisted on pressing on. That clouded the first part of the trip but You brought us safely through and we enjoyed ourselves once we got there. We picked up dinner and Lee rented a video that we watched together before bed.

The next day, we went out and shared a breakfast (I don't need a separate one since my appetite is still not back up to normal. I am now down to 125 lbs. from my original 156 "before-stroke" weight.)

We browsed stores with beautiful stained glass and Lee bought me earrings with a picture of seagulls flying over a beautiful, blue ocean. We also got a beautiful stained glass angel to suspend from the foyer ceiling at Christmas. It was a nice day that felt like playing hooky from any cares that being home might bring. It's good to do that every now and then. I enjoyed the ride back home more after I put my faith in You to bring us safely back despite the concerns I have over Lee's driving. I decided to direct my thoughts toward his well being rather than my own and that changed my whole attitude. Thank you, Lord. Let me continue to focus on the needs of others but only be concerned about what I can control. AMEN

11/8/03

Thank you, Lord. Yesterday, I received a called confirming that I had been selected to participate in the Pepper study... HALLELUJAH! My progress had dropped off because I was no longer exercising as I used to. Now, I will be motivated to start again. Before I can give them a start date, however, I have to wait to see when the doctor can schedule my gall bladder surgery. It seems that everything is picking up at once, now that we're getting nearer the holidays.

I woke up this morning concerned about Mother's move and the availability of people to help or if I can even be there to participate. I reminded myself that You will take care of it and that I should do the part of it that I can control and have faith that the rest will be done. So I will lay out the floor plan and furniture arrangement we agreed upon as a guide for the movers that day. That will be a fun part to do. Then I will check on the availability of people to help that day and make sure they all have directions. Lee has a video job that day and Everett has school. Finally, I will ask Michele to be in charge of directing folks (she's good at that). Thank you Lord for laying it out for me.

11/9/03

Thank You God for speaking to me this morning and making another thing clear. The thing that stands out the most is the fact that I am still *me* with just a few things I have temporarily forgotten how to do. I can still do most of the things I used to do around the house as long as I listen to my body and take a break or switch to another task when I feel the need.

The things I have been trying to do for others to prove to myself that I'm still the "same old me" were unnecessary. And feeling guilty has no benefit at all. *GUILT IS THE HIGH PRICE PAID FOR WHICH I GET NO RETURN ON MY PAYMENT.* Then, I end up resenting the person for whom I could not do the activity (when it was my idea in the first place). How confusing it must be to deal with me. Thank you, Father, for being so patient and for surrounding me with people who love me enough to tolerate strange attitudes until I get the words from You that straighten me out.

It is said that, until we learn from our actions, we are destined to repeat them. I know that I have said this somewhere before in this journal but this time I will try to remember to take it to heart. All of my energy and creativity for awhile will now be directed toward helping Lee make this house more livable instead of trying to project my ideas onto Mother's house. Lee has hinted toward this when I suggested decorating Mother's new apartment and he said, "Why don't you decorate this one?" I have used the excuse that I know he can decorate better, but could that just be an excuse for unwillingness to take on a task that I would have to finish?

Sometimes I find myself contentedly saying that I really don't have to do anything, that I can just leave beds unmade, dust building up, or dishes unwashed because I don't want to overtire myself and Lee will not get mad. How lazy and uncaring can I be? I say I love him but I'm letting him carry his load and mine, doubling up on his video work to make up for my lack of income, planning and cooking all the meals, doing all the yard work, and cleaning and reorganizing the inside of the house.

Thank you for the eye opener, Lord, and I pray that You will guide me to begin *doing* without *overdoing*. Let me plan my work and work my plan still cognizant of what my body is telling me and listening closely to you. I thank you again for Lee, Lord, and help me do this without guilt. As Maya Angelou once said, "I did then what I knew to do. Now that I know better, I'll do better." AMEN

11/11/03- Losing My Mind?

Did something happen to my mind and no one is letting me know? Sometimes I feel very sure that I've made the right decision about something only to be equally as sure later that the exact opposite is true. On thinking about Mother's move, I know that it is something we started together and are both looking forward to. Why, then, have I balked at the prospect of being involved? Would I not be hurt if everyone tried to eliminate me from the joy of seeing it through? And am I not most happy when I feel I am in charge of something? Why, then, is the very prospect of someone counting on me making me feel overwhelmed?

I seem to be complaining about it more than anyone else, and when they back off and Mother says that I don't have to do anything, that she would like it if I was just there, then the threat of being overwhelmed seems to subside and I want to be involved again. How confusing it must be to those around me. One day I hope to be able to explain to them how confused I was inside without really knowing how irrational my behavior was. So I think right now that I will do the things I can do by phone today (making sure the phone is hooked up, the mail is switched, etc.) and that everyone had directions to both houses for Saturday.

I will make arrangements to be picked up and taken to the new apartment and leave the move to the guys. I will also make sure that Weldon is renting the truck. Most of all, I will eliminate the words, "*in charge*" from of my vocabulary and actions. We are all adults and no one has to order others around. Help me, Father, to stick to that rule most of all. They (and I) will love me more if I just blend in as part of the team, doing the part of it I love to do.

Please help them forgive me, Father, for being such a pain. I know that You just told me that it is already done. I have no need to even talk about it anymore. I will just let my actions speak for me. I won't feel guilt, just love, toward those who forgive so readily. Thank you for giving me this time to speak with You and for always being there patiently waiting until I come to my senses. And thanks for Lee, hovering in the background, just being there when he can help make my life a little easier and more pleasant. You must love me an awful lot to give me so much. Thank you, Lord.

11/16/03

I'm up and writing at about 5:30 this morning, having gone to bed just a little earlier last night. Both Lee and I were tired from getting to bed after 1:30 the night before because of videotaping a concert with the Extensions of Faith choir. I helped out at the table selling tapes. Then, Lee had a wedding on Saturday and I was up good and early to be picked up by Heather to go and help Mother move into her brand new apartment.

It was a little chaotic at first with people getting their signals crossed in regard to where they should be at which time, but, together, we pulled it off and all went home feeling tired but happy. Mother was in awe of how much bigger this place seems to be as compared to her old place. She even forgot it was hers for a minute when we were about to leave and she wrapped up a donut to take "home" with her.

We feel so much better about her living there, surrounded by other seniors who have built in alarm systems if she needs them. I had stressed out over who was going to handle all the many facets of the move but when I finally "*let go and let God do it*", everything turned out just fine. I found that even when people did not want to take the lead in getting things done, they would if I didn't try to take the responsibility. I will have to remember to commend everyone on their efforts. It was even enjoyable at some points as we all pulled together. I found that with everyone doing whatever they saw needed to be done and only giving suggestions when asked, it all melded together beautifully. Another lesson learned.

Day before yesterday, I was in touch with the Pepper Study people trying to schedule a start date, only to find that they can't provide the transportation that they had promised. I thought about not participating after all, not wanting Lee to have to take me 3 times a week. When I told him, he reminded me that we have transportation. It was then that I realized that the improvement in my ability to do things would be a blessing to my loved ones as well as to me.

So I will call them back tomorrow and schedule a start date. Then I'll talk to everyone who might be able to get me there (Department of Aging, Senior Cab program, Mike, Michelle, etc.) I may even find someone to carpool with. Who knows? I am a "find a way or make a way" person and this is too important to let slip by. Thank you, Lord, for determination.

11/23/03

It is really hard to believe that another year has almost passed. It has been a year that I wouldn't have traded for anything because I have never experienced so much love in my entire life. As it grows closer to the holidays, it seems that Lee is working even harder to make sure that new and beautiful things are surrounding me. Yesterday, he hung two stained glass Angel panels we had selected at Costco in front of the side kitchen window where I can see them first thing in the morning. He has been busy cleaning and decorating parts of the house in spite of the extra load he has taken on producing more videotapes for people to share with their loved ones for the holidays. I love him so much and just thank You God for the gift of him.

Thank You, also, for Michele who showed me such a fun time yesterday when she took me to the mall to shop for a new nightie for the hotel I'm taking Lee to for his birthday.

The Westin in NJ is famous for its "Heavenly beds" and "Heavenly showers" and I want to be pleasing to his sight after wearing mostly flannel pajamas since the stroke. I pray that he really enjoys himself and that I really won't push for feelings of intimacy but let everything flow naturally.

We were able to get a motorized scooter in the mall and I had high time eating free cookies in the Christmas store, Godiva chocolate Michele bought me while riding down the mall, and laughing like crazy as I tried to maneuver the scooter in and out of tight places without taking out any walls (or any toes). People were so patient and in good humor about it.

One thing that has truly amazed me since this stroke is just how nice and considerate people are to those who are disabled. I will definitely remember to pass that on when I am no longer disabled.

I awoke this morning considering whether to leave all earning ideas go and just truly enjoy all the fun part of this season. It is a tempting idea but I think that Michelle is counting on me to do some holiday selling with her. So I will mingle the two things, working our joint business, doing the faces of the ladies who have influenced my life since the stroke, and spending a Spa Day with Michelle and Debbie. I plan to attend every holiday function that I can and really make the most out of this season. Thank You Lord for the opportunity. AMEN

11/27/03- THANKSGIVING

This was the first Thanksgiving that I can remember during my married life that we were away from the family. But it was a blessed one, spent with Michele's extended family up at Rita's loving, welcoming home in NJ. There were 11 of us —Michele, Everett, Cameron, Ethan, Keren, Greg, Regina, Caleb, Rita, Lee, and Me. I said grace and asked for your blessing on us but didn't say all that I wanted because I didn't want to become emotional and didn't want to make the prayer too long. I just wanted to express how grateful I was that You allowed me to live to see another Thanksgiving surrounded by loving family and friends. But You knew what was in my heart and I'm so glad.

I planned for those two days up there to

be extra special for Lee because it was part of his birthday celebration. But, following Your example, he always gives more than he receives and made it extra special for me as well. We went straight to the Princeton Westin hotel and tried out their famous "heavenly bed" with enough fluffy covers to encompass me and remind me of the quilts Mama used to cover me with when I stayed down the country. We had a great dinner at Rita's even though she kept apologizing for looking like Rerun with her French beret and casual clothes.

Instead, she focused on making us feel loved and welcome. I had to go back to the hotel earlier than I would have in the past because my energy level has not yet returned, but no one seemed to mind. I had Michele pick up the red nightgown that we had looked at when we went to the mall. I even brought the bottle of wine and the wineglasses and candle that I had originally packed for our planned Valentine's Day get-away before the stroke. But I let good sense take over that night and, realizing that I would be forcing myself to act romantic and trying to stay awake, I slipped into my silk pajamas and kissed Lee goodnight.

We both thoroughly enjoyed all the romantic preparation the following night after having a fun day to ourselves, starting with going out to breakfast, riding around in the rain, napping, shopping and having ice cream and hot lemonade while listening to carolers sing, then showering in the "heavenly shower", and going to the movies. It is much better not to force things to fit into a planned schedule. Lee always manages to make the occasion special for me and I'm so grateful.

Those two days at the hotel almost made me feel like my old self instead of the "dependent" person that I have a tendency to feel like since the stroke. I pray that I will be strong enough to not let that feeling overtake me. I know that, with Your help, I will be able to bounce back. Thank you, Lord. AMEN

12/05/03- The First Snow of the Season!!!

It's funny. I think it snowed about this same time last year... and snowed, and snowed, and snowed until about March. Yet, I can't contain my excitement when I see that first fluffy accumulation on the holly bushes and trees outside the windows. Thank you Jesus that I can still have the wonder of seeing things through my "child" eyes. It helps to add to that wonder, the relief at not having to worry about how Mother is going to get to dialysis today.

You provided us with a helper, right on time, who seems to be everything that we need. She has a 4-wheel drive vehicle and doesn't mind driving in bad weather, is willing to be there on dialysis mornings to fix Mother some breakfast, wrap her arm, and take her to dialysis on time. Then she will pick her up, bring her home, prepare her a snack, and fix her dinner. I know that she must be a gift from you because she appeared just after Mother fell and fractured her pelvis and was advised to stay in the wheelchair for 6 weeks.

The bus that was taking her to dialysis was not equipped to carry a wheelchair so you sent us Becky Carpenter. Thank you, Lord. Between her and Alicia who comes on Tuesdays and Thursdays when Mother doesn't go to dialysis and provides the lightness and joy of decorating for Christmas, taking Mother out or going to the store for her, it seems that we have all that we need to make Mother's life more pleasant. Add to that the camaraderie she can have with the other seniors who also just moved into her building, it seems that there is an ideal environment for her. Please let it be all that we hope for and more. Bless her Lord because she has sacrificed all her adult life to be a blessing to us. AMEN

12/09/03

You know how the small things can mean so much more than a fabulous gift? Well, that's the way it was today. When I got up, I started feeling the irresistible urge to get out and just go somewhere; no place special but just to run around, browse, snack, and maybe buy a few things. A trip to Costco came to mind where I could move about freely in the motorized cart, looking at Christmas displays, snacking on free samples, and be greeted and hugged by old friends.

When I suggested to Lee that we just go out to let me cash my checks and maybe pick up a few things, his first reaction was that he had a lot to do. I know that is true because several people have requested copies of their videotapes for Christmas and Lee is still trying to fix things in the house. But after Michele came by and I told her how I felt the need to get out and she couldn't take me, Lee stopped what he was doing and suggested that I go with him because he had some things to pick up. He took me to the bank and then to Costco where I had a wonderful time riding around free. We looked at displays together and unrushed and then, after being there a couple of hours, I even got a hotdog and soda and came home happy and tired and took a nap.

He is so wonderful to me Lord. He even got copies of the pictures I wanted to send to Wayne and I'm ashamed to say that my first thought was of putting them in an album for Wayne, not remembering until later that I had thought of doing that for Lee weeks ago. Sometimes I wonder where my head is but I'm so glad that you gave me the gift of afterthought. Please help me to keep my priorities straight and remember the one whom I love most. Thank you, Lord. AMEN

12/12/03- Spa Day!

Thank you, Lord for a day of relaxation, prayer, and rejuvenation as You allowed Debbie, Michelle, and me to take time out of this busy season to forget about the hustle and bustle and making money, and spend a fun day together. How blessed it was! We had not seen Debbie in over a year and we were able to spend hours just catching up. We went to the spa for relaxing massages, followed by a quiet time in the relaxation room, surrounded by soft music, a fire in the fireplace, cool drinking water and fresh fruit, with aroma-therapy wraps around our necks.

We enjoyed laughing and talking while we got dressed and then walked right next door into the Atlanta Bread Co. where we had delicious clam chowder and a special holiday sandwich of turkey, cranberries, lettuce and tomato on special bread. DELICIOUS! We sat at a window, completely unrushed by anyone there, and Debbie blessed us with one of her special prayers. Sharing pictures and stories of the families was just what we needed and, when we left the restaurant, You blessed us by letting us spot the Home Store which none of us had ever visited before.

What a time we had, delighting over the beautiful and reasonably priced items in each aisle. We all did some shopping, laughing as we helped each other with some selections. When I began to tire, we all agreed to return home, and we took a picture together in my living room. That day, I really spread joy, as it radiated from inside me. Thank you, Lord, for the joy of that day. May I continue to share that feeling throughout the season and throughout the year? AMEN

12/17/03- Colonoscopy

Thank you, Lord, for bringing me safely through today's procedure with good results. Doctors thought that the pain I had experienced might have been because of some obstruction in my colon since I was having difficulty with regular bowel movements, but the test showed that my colon was clear. Now we have eliminated one more thing and I'm grateful.

As it grows closer and closer to Christmas, my favorite time of the year, I can't seem to get in that same frame of mind. Even though I had Mike pick up the gift for Lee that he had mentioned that he wanted, I don't look forward to giving it to him. I would like to have given him something that I actually created, like the album I thought of earlier, but it would require someone else select it or take me out looking for it and then help me put it together.

Michele had offered but she has so much to do and has already taken out the time to create beautiful holly swags for our doors, showed me a wonderful time when she took me to the mall to select a gown when we were going away for Lee's birthday, created a centerpiece and display for Mother, and still did the things she needed to do with the boys. She has such a good heart but Lord, sometimes I feel so frustrated at not being able to do for myself and those whom I helped in the past.

Lee has continued to shoulder his tasks as well as mine, making sure that I want for nothing and still trying to keep up extra video work to keep finances at an even keel. I'm afraid that he will get worn out and then, who will help out? I am getting the answer even as I write this Lord. I see how I am trying to figure it out without adding You into the equation and that could never work out.

I should do the part of it I love to do (spreading joy among my loved ones, something the world seems to be in short supply of right now).   I should also *stop concentrating on lack, counting instead, all the blessings You have showered down on me* --being able to walk without the wheelchair, Lee and I doing the Christmas cards together, a clean report from the colonoscopy, Mother and me still alive to celebrate another Christmas, Lee still alive and loving me in spite of the fact that at least 4 of my friends have lost their husbands within the past year. HOW BLESSED I AM!!! Thanks Lord, for this talk.

I know now that it is time to get on about my Father's work ... spreading JOY. The first place I'll start is reigniting the flame within me. It's impossible to spread the flame if I'm letting mine flicker out. The real joy of the season is in remembering the great gift You gave to the world but I have not focused on that lately. I will go back among Your people where I can be reminded, instead of trying to keep this flame burning alone. I feel the enemy's demons constantly trying to douse it and I know that

I need You, Lord. to protect it and me. Help me Jesus. I thank you. Now it will be all right. AMEN

12/20/03—Depression

This morning I'm writing this from memory because I didn't choose to write as I was going through it. I am feeling much better this morning with a new outlook on life, so it is easier to talk about it. I think it is important to record this because I may need to read over it later to see how You brought me through it. I hope that talking about it doesn't put me back in a funk with the stress causing my ulcer to act up again. Lord, please help me to divorce myself emotionally from these feelings as I write this. You are telling me that it is all right to go with my feelings and I'll trust You to bring me back up out of that valley when I'm through writing. This is the way I recall my feelings:

I don't know what's happening to me. The least little thing sets me to crying again, almost like it was right after I had my stroke. Mike was just talking to me on the phone, asking if I had been able to straighten out the issue with the bank where I had overdrawn my account and he offered to put money in the bank for me. Then I started crying and couldn't talk to him anymore. He said he loved me and I just hung up without saying anymore. I wanted to escape and cry where Lee couldn't hear me (it makes him feel helpless when I cry and he can't do anything to help. He is working day and night to do things to make me happy).

I went to the bathroom and prayed that Mike wouldn't call him but he did because he was worried. Lee came to the bathroom door and asked me what was the matter and I said "nothing", trying to sound convincing. He asked why I was stressing Mike out if nothing was wrong and I didn't answer. I tried to stifle my sobs with a towel after he left the door and decided to take a shower so the water might muffle the sound. I knew that he did not go back down to his office even though he was working hard to fill the requests from his video clients.

I stayed in the shower as long as I could, trying not to sob out loud and then came out, determined to talk to Lee after I got into my night clothes about what was happening to my emotions. I recalled Michele telling me about a bout with depression after Ethan was born and how she finally gave in and went to speak to the doctor about it. She took medication for several months and then was better. None of us was aware of what she was going through but I thank God that she was wise enough to seek help in time.

I decided that I would do the same but feared that Lee, having seen the same thing happen to his Mother, might try to protect me from doctors who tend to over medicate people, and might try to discourage me from seeking help. Isn't it funny how we play out these scenarios in our heads, taking both sides of the conversation; how often we give the enemy an opportunity to sneak in and send us onto the wrong path?

I then shifted the blame to Mother who, earlier that day had asked me to go along with her and her aide down to see Dr. Ord, the cancer specialist. When I had said that I couldn't but did not give a reason, she said that I "just didn't want to". Then I felt guilty and that triggered stress.

Michele had talked to me about stressing out and blamed Mother for asking me to do things that she knew I shouldn't (or couldn't) do. She now has enough hired (and volunteer) help that she shouldn't need anything else, but old habits die hard. I realize now that I should take Mother's requests for help the same way I might if some other patient at the hospital had asked; I would love to be able to do it, but feel no guilt that both of us are in the same state of being unable to help the other right now. It won't last always and meanwhile we'll both concentrate on getting stronger.

Michele had said that she or Cat was planning to speak to Mother regarding this but I prayed on it and spoke to Mother myself.

I printed out all the information she needed along with phone numbers and told her that I had gone through two stress-related incidents within the past two weeks; one of which had sent me to the hospital, and that I felt unable to handle any decisions or help with anyone else's problems for awhile. I asked her not to call me for solutions or to discuss problems with me for awhile. She said that she might mention it without thinking, and I told her that I probably would just not answer her calls for awhile. She suggested that I just call her when I felt like talking. I agreed.

I did not call her the following day and night and by evening, when it was time for Date Night, my ulcer started giving me stomach pains so bad that I decided to stay home. Lee didn't put up a fuss and I settled down to a TV movie while Lee continued to decorate beautifully all around me. I got up to do a little something, but when my stomach started to ache again, I settled back in. My stomach had eased off by bedtime and I awoke this morning, feeling better and with a much better outlook and plans for "love gifts" to give at Christmas. I was feeling badly about giving gifts that others had to pick out and pay for with just payback promises from me.

So now, I thank you, God, for letting me come through the recall of this "valley period" feeling better. I will carry out my plans as best I can and, most of all, see or talk to Mother and try to help her understand that she is not to blame for the changes in my brain. Help me to say it right Lord and let her still feel loved. And thanks again for the love of family, especially Lee. AMEN

12/28/03-1/05/04- What A Blessing—Right On Time!

We went on our long-awaited trip to Disney World (Michele, Everett, Cameron, Ethan, Keren, Lee, and I). Everyone but Lee and I drove down together in a van. Lee and I flew and got there in 2 hours. The doctor had given me samples of pills to try to calm my stress but I think just getting away from the situation helped tremendously. What a time we had! The condo that Karen Underwood had let us use was on Disney property and was beautiful. It had a full kitchen, a King sized wrought iron bed in a large master bedroom with louvered shutters opening into the master bathroom overlooking a Jacuzzi. There was a separate glassed-in shower in another room and even a separate room for the toilet. The living room had a sofa bed and TV and there was also a dining room and deck. *Fabulous*! One of the things that I loved most, though, was the scooter that was delivered to the condo shortly after we arrived. It was brand new, with a red velvet seat and gave me the independence to get around by myself (Thank *you, Jesus!)* something that I had not experienced for almost a year since the stroke.

This allowed me to have quiet time to commune with You without anyone waiting to move me to the next place or having to feel guilty about leaving me by myself when I was too tired to keep up the busy schedule the others had planned. Instead, I woke up and leisurely did my stretches, dressed, took my breakfast bagel and juice, and got on my scooter and rode down to have breakfast by the pier.

I enjoyed watching the ducks and seagulls and feeling the warmth of near-80-degree sunshine warm my bones and lift my spirit. Another day, I rode around the walkways of the condo, through the quiet paths surrounding a lake and past beautiful flowering gardens under blue skies. I rode over a bridge that connected the condo to the boardwalk on the other side of the water and enjoyed exploring a few shops. I picked up a few items (bread, bagels, and peanut butter) and even went into a candy store where I selected several kinds of candy that Lee and I like. What freedom!

One of my most memorable times was when I took breakfast down to the beach and, because I had the scooter, I could take off my brace and shoes, sit in a porch swing that they had on the beach, and just dig my toes in the warm sand. Heaven! I had to call Cat from there just to let her hear the joy in my voice. I had a chance to feed the seagulls shrimp and potato chips from that same swing before we left for home at the end of our vacation.

We enjoyed great times together with the gang, as well, seeing the joy on Cameron's face and Ethan saying, "I didn't like that ride" after getting off a ride in Disneyworld. But they both enjoyed riding with me on my scooter, one on my knee and the other on the back. We even had the chance to keep them overnight in our condo and take them to breakfast on the boardwalk the next morning; riding the ferry, swimming and playing in the sand and hot tub. What a life!

Lee showed his love and care even more, if that is possible. He made sure that my scooter was always in position to go before he left, and still made me know that I was desirable, taking showers and Jacuzzi baths together, playing beautiful music that he brought and letting our passion flow with massages I had longed for since before the stroke. How can I help but love that man? Thank you, God for the gift of him.

1/6/2004- MY NAME IS CECELIA – I AM AN ENABLER...

I can finally face the fact that I have two choices; I can either stop trying to solve Mother's everyday problems voluntarily and live at home OR I can be forced to stop by living in a hospital. The strain on my brain has delayed my ability to focus on my stroke recovery and has me stressed to the point where I am taking an additional medication daily and thinking of contacting a psychiatrist to ease the crying outbursts.

The only doctor I need to rely on is Doctor Jesus and since I know He is always there, I need to focus more on helping myself after He gives me guidance and earthly helpers. He blessed me with Lee who constantly does all the things he thinks I need to help me recover, even to the point of doing some of the things I would do for Mother if I were able. God also gave me Michele who stepped in to supply Mother's needs in ways I couldn't even when I was well (finding helpers, cooking dishes, creating decorations, etc.). He also provided the help of Michael, Cat, Byron, Thelma, Jerome, Carol, and two weekly aides who have all stepped in whenever Mother needed something…9 people who took my place…yet Mother continues to call to ask for my help or the help of Lee.

It is time for me to take charge of my life and my emotions with God's help. I know it will not be easy because of the long-ingrained guilt factor, but I know that with God's help, I can do it one step at a time. Some of the steps I will take are as follows:

Begin meditation, prayer, and exercising again on a daily basis

Let the answering machine take all my calls and return only those I need to respond to at a set time each day

Don't volunteer anyone else's services.

Only ask for help after I have thought through a task and attempted it 3 times

As much as possible, arrange all appointments or errands to coincide with errands a person has to run

Take advantage of the offer by Michele or Mike to take me places I need to go once per week

WITH THE HELP OF GOD, I WILL BE ABLE TO ACHIEVE THIS

1/8/03

I am up writing this at 4 a.m. after being awake since about 3. We got back late Monday night and, on Tuesday morning, Mother had already called me to ask for one of the numbers I had put on the list that I gave her. She said she had an appointment and was not sure how she would get there. She asked if Lee could take her. When I made an excuse not to ask him, she took a cab but complained that she was running out of vouchers instead of sending for more. I found myself just wanting to sleep all day, taking two naps and still fighting sleep at 8:00 at night.

I awoke this morning wrestling with ways to help her since her helpers are both dealing with sickness right now, but now that I think of it, so am I. Help me Lord to read over my resolutions 3 times or more each day and to stick by them. Thank you Lord. You know I love her but I can't help her until I help me.

This morning's entry in my *Daily Guidepost* listing things that mattered to the writer led me to thinking about my list.

Things That Matter To Me
(*And Make Me Thank God*)

My husband, Lee's, arm over me
with his body snuggled close

Waking up to blue sunshiny skies

Snowflakes falling

The hush of my morning walk when I
can't even hear my own footsteps

Crunching through fallen leaves

The smell of the woods

Squirrels standing on their hind legs eating
bits of food from their front paws

Tiny chipmunks standing up like miniature
squirrels, filling their cheeks to bursting

The new blooms on the hibiscus
bushes in my Prayer garden

Quiet, peaceful water of a pond
surrounded by wildflowers

Waves rolling gently in to the shore

Sun rising over the ocean spreading beams across

the sky, outlining clouds in iridescent orange

*Sunset over the ocean like a brilliant orange
ball shooting rays out over the waves*

*A field of wildflowers with more
shades of color than you can count*

The sound of birds singing in the morning

First flowers of Spring

Autumn-colored trees

The smell of fresh-cut grass

*Lee, lovingly caring for our yard,
creating a thing of beauty*

*Lying back on the chaise lounge on
a warm day, just "being"*

*Sipping a fresh fruit smoothie
lovingly made by Lee*

*Feeding seagulls as they swoop
and call to each other*

*The feel of sand between my toes as I
dig my bare feet down into it*

Swinging on a porch swing

Writing in my journal as I talk with You, Lord

A moving gospel song that brings
back warm memories

Riding unhurried with windows open along a
tree-lined road and listening to soft background
music selected by Lee just for such occasions

Hearing the "aromatherapy" music
and feeling Lee's loving, strong hands
give me a massage as only he can

For These And All Things, Father, I
Thank You For Lovingly Giving Me.

Just as I thought I might be getting a handle on my stress, these things happed in one week:

1/10/04   Mother went to hospital- hardly able to walk//tongue feeling like it was swelling—numbness in right hand

1/14/04 Cat's husband, Cliff, taken to Sinai hospital—severe chest pain – aorta about to burst—transported to hospital

1/15/04   stint measured for and ordered—surgery scheduled for Tuesday

1/16/04 Mother went to rehab

1/17/04   Cliff transferred out of intensive care to regular room

1/18/04 Cliff passed at 5:00 a.m.

1/28/04   *LAZY, COMFORTABLE, COMPLACENT—*

Completely undetected by me, these traits had taken over the real me. I had been praying to God to restore my body and my exuberant personality and all the while these things had been creeping in and taking over. Upon awakening this morning at 8:45, I took a good look at myself in the mirror. I had a wrinkle across the side of my face from lying too long on the pillow and had even thought about just lying there luxuriating just a little longer looking at the beauty of the snow and ice and telling myself that I really didn't have to move. Lee would understand if I needed more rest. *Rest from what?*

He was already up and working in his office, trying to catch up with his tape orders before the next video job came in. Yesterday, he had worked at it all day and still found time to go out in the icy conditions with his bandaged foot wrapped in plastic to try to find ways to keep air from coming under the front door. He went out again to get us fresh fruit and even to pick up something for dinner. Meanwhile, I was telling Mike that I had spoiled Lee by making chicken and dumplings the day before (the first from-scratch meal in a year!) I had gotten to the place where I had convinced myself that I should stop and sit or lie down whenever I felt tired or sleepy. It wasn't the overwork that caused the stroke. It was more likely the stress that I let myself experience in thinking of things I *should have done* rather than listing them and accomplishing as many as I could.

I often tell Cat that that is the way to go but not practicing what I preach. *But that was before today*. Thank you God for opening my eyes. Today, I will put in place a living list of the things I need to accomplish, when I am sitting down and when moving around. When I feel weary of one type, I will change to the other. And whenever I feel tired, I will do 15 minutes more of one task from the other list. Help me Lord to accomplish this without fear of hurting myself. Thank you Lord. AMEN

2/3/04- The 1st Anniversary of My New Life - look Where He's Brought Me From

I can hardly believe that it has been a year since that fateful day. I can truly say that I'm a survivor and I couldn't have done it without all of the love and support from God, Lee, family and friends. A year ago, I could not:

1. speak clearly

2. breathe except in small gasps

3. swallow without thinking

4. sit up unaided

5. walk

6. move my right arm, leg, or foot

After 5 days in North Arundel Hospital, almost a month at Kernan being rehabilitated, and outpatient therapy along with my own exercises, I can now:

1. walk with or without the cane, sometimes without the brace

2. raise my right arm while lying on my back

3. move my fingers (not always on command)

4. speak fairly clearly though sometimes my lips get numb preventing clear speech—also not as loud

5. breathe normally

6. right foot still doesn't bend or move toes on command

7. Help others problem solve about 70% of the time

With a stress tab once/day, not crying sporadically

I am still taking naps daily, though it is now down to one 1-hour nap per day. All in all I am doing well, although I have had times during the year when I wondered if I made the right decision in not letting them give me the tPA which might have reversed the effects of the stroke. But then I think that instead of Mike calling like he did tonight to wish me a happy anniversary of the year since the stroke. Lee and the kids could have been sad today as they commemorated the one-year anniversary of my death had the drug had adverse effects. I thank you God that I am still here. AMEN

2/4/04—It Has Been a Wonderful Day. Thank You Lord.

I've just got to stop and say thank you, Lord for the multiple blessings You have given us between yesterday and today. They are:

1. Michele called to say that she left a message on Becky's (Mother's helper) answering machine telling her what a dilemma she left us in by not responding to calls stating what her intentions were for working with Mother and driving her to dialysis. Today, Becky not only called but also stopped by, we reached an agreement and she promises to start back to work on Monday. Thank you, Jesus.

2. Mike called to say that they had effortlessly sold their present home for more than they

expected and that today, they are the proud owners of a new hole in the ground where their new home is about to be built. Thank you, Lord.

3. Cat called and said that she had resolved some major financial obstacles by herself, resulting in a $25,000 savings on a loan owed, finding a way to get money credited to her bills that Cliff had left in his account, and setting up automatic payments for her life and health insurance. She also enrolled with a recommended grief counselor in her area. Hallelujah!

4. I was given my schedule for therapy sessions for the Pepper Study and was able to line up rides for all six weeks with the exception of Fridays. I will ask Lee to do those and that way; we can start Date Night even earlier. Thank you for Tricia McDaniel, a 20-year stroke survivor, who has volunteered to drive as a way of thanks to you for giving her back that ability. Please help

me to remember to use that as an example and pass it on. AMEN

2/5/04- LIKE A TON OF BRICKS

Sometimes God has to send something that hits you like a 2X4 or a ton of bricks in order to get your attention. That is what happened to me tonight with a simple question that was on the form I was filling out to try to justify why I was not yet working anywhere since my stroke one year ago. It simply asked me to list my daily activities. It stopped me cold when I tried to think of what constructive things I did all day and could not honestly come up with any. Yet, I am always worn out by naptime at 2 and well ready to go to bed before 11. Could it be boredom? I am acting like some of those welfare Mothers who I always said I couldn't imagine being like, sitting around waiting for their monthly welfare check. Now I have almost slipped into that same mode.

Lee deserves a medal for putting up with this attitude for such a long time but sometimes it is easier to let a person see herself as she really is. Lesson learned! Lord, please help me make a change, beginning tomorrow and improving each day. Help me to remember not to try to make too many changes at once, but to work diligently on one at a time. Thank you Lord. AMEN

2/21/04- My Accomplishments

It is 11:20 p.m. and I am bone tired and sleepy but I couldn't go to bed without thanking you for helping me to stick to it until I accomplished more toward my goal. Monday, I asked for your help in laying out my goals to once again work my Mary Kay business, but this time, with a business plan. I don't intend to wait on others to do it with me, though I do plan to share information along the way to those you bring my way. Today was an especially good day in which I accomplished:

1. Washing 2 loads of clothes

2. Drying and folding 3 loads

3. Preparing and eating 2 of my meals

4. Creating a flyer for the unit contest

5. Modifying my customer list and sending out flyers to about 18 people (to expand my customer base and get orders)

6. Sold $95 in product to a client

7. Sold my first new moisturizer in advance of ordering it and had my first client agree to be a part of skincare panel (Only 12 more moisturizers to go to be in company contest)

8. Left my office and spare room straight

9. Took only one half-hour nap

10. Cleaned face and teeth before bed

11. Washed dinner dishes

12. Cleaned washer and dryer tops

13. Moved vacuum out of laundry room into workroom

14. Returned Rita's call

15. Spoke to Mother several times and congratulated her on her accomplishments

Thank you Lord for giving me the strength to persevere. AMEN

2/27/04- The Storm is Passing Over

Lord, let me not forget or lose the passion I felt during the midst of the storm. This morning as I came into the spare room to get dressed, I heard a bird calling from the tree just outside my window. I quickly opened the blinds to try to get in position to catch a glimpse of him, but God, You put him on the highest branch so that I could easily see him. Then another bird joined him which made me start to give You thanks, but the more I thanked you the more You sent.

A beautiful red cardinal soon joined them and began eating old berries off of the tree, and just as I was thinking that this was a sure sign of the coming of Spring, You sent me my first Robin of the year. Thank you Jesus. It brought tears to my eyes and words of praise to my lips. No matter how rough the winter, You help us to weather it with the knowledge that "this, too, shall pass". We can always count on you. And then You whispered those words to my spirit, "the storm is passing over" and I knew that You were not only talking about the season, but my struggle.

Just as I know that the sunny days will begin to lengthen now and the flowers will bloom once again to increase my joy, my body will begin to strengthen and I will once again bring You joy. I will empty myself so that You may fill me up as I continue on my mission to *spread joy*. AMEN

3/1/04- THANK YOU GOD...

For this weekend when Mike came to pick up Mother and me to take us to do whatever we wanted to do in 3-4 hours. We went to see the building of his new home, which is now almost two stories done. Then we toured the model and it is fabulous. We followed that with lunch at the outdoor umbrella tables at Checkers. Thank you for the warmth of the sunshine and the blue skies. It warmed our souls and rejuvenated our spirits. We had fun bopping to the beat of the oldies playing over the speakers while the three of us laughed and had lunch together.

Mike went to pick up some small things we needed from the store and Mother said it felt like old times as the two of us enjoyed each other's company. We topped the day off by surprising Mother with a stop at Mikie's, our favorite ice cream store where we each got our favorite kind. We knew it was a special blessing because they rarely have them both in at the same time. Mike brought us home to enjoy a much-needed nap after a wonderful day. Thank you Lord for him, for Mother's happiness, and for the joy inside of me.

The happiness continued the next day when Lee took me to join Cat and her grandkids to surprise Hattie who was preaching the sermon at her church. We were welcomed with open arms. Thank you for inspiring me to take pencils, colored paper and treats to have the girls draw something they heard or saw in church. They presented Hattie with the drawings following her sermon and she was really pleased. We all had lunch afterwards at the church and I managed to sneak in another short nap after Lee reminded me that we were invited to a surprise party for a member of his volleyball team.

I knew that I had to place my Mary Kay

order first because You had inspired me to invite my friends who agreed to try the new moisturizer (mainly because I asked them to, I'm sure) to come over for a pampering deep-cleansing session so we can all start the moisturizer together. It should be great fun. Thank you for blessing me with 18 of the 20 whom I asked in the last week.

Thanks, also for the call from Reva, the nurse at Kernan, who has asked 12 nurses and aides who were as good to me while I was hospitalized, to join us for a makeover session. I hope that they will come here and let me welcome them into my home. I also thank you for the blessing of the therapists who are scheduled to come here this evening for makeovers along with the lady I met last night at the party. You are truly blessing me Lord and I pray that I keep this perspective of treating them out of gratitude because they have truly had a wondrous impact on my life. Thank you for opening my eyes and my heart. AMEN

4/27/04

It has been a while since my last entry and lots of wonderful and sometimes not so wonderful things have happened for me. I will start with the most recent while it is fresh in my mind and catch up later when I get a chance.

Yesterday, for the first time in my 13-year Mary Kay career, I finally saw the financial rewards of my earnings! Yes, I have certainly received lots of money from this career from time to time ($1000-dollar days, $848 commissions, etc.), but this was the result of planning, dividing money the way Mary Kay teaches, and actually having the money that is to be paid to me, guilt-free, as my paycheck. Best of all, I know that I can repeat the process and recreate it again and again. Hallelujah! I have found the key. And, to make sure that I have the discipline, I will start to do it again, not waiting 3 months this time, but paying myself after a month. I have requested that Loretta allow me to share this lesson with the group at our next meeting and I will have my material prepared ahead of time to help them understand. Thank You, Lord, for this glorious feeling of accomplishment and the need to share it, not for my glory but for the benefit of those who need it.

Best of all, I felt no need to exaggerate the numbers to make them more impressive. You gave me a talent to see what I would make of it and when I show that I can use that one to its maximum, You will make me Stewart over more things. Right now, all that I have is all that I need. Please strengthen my willpower to make this happen again and again. This time, I will save it, untouched, for a month and shorten periods between pays until it becomes bi-weekly.

Meanwhile, I'll act responsibly in spending my $600+ that is awaiting me in the bank. I will track my spending of this seed money; some being allotted to the fund that the children and grandchildren of Mother set up to keep her finances going. I will also begin to pay back a debt a little at a time and gradually take over payment of my own expenses. I will always remember to tithe first, to New Psalmist or Cherry Hill Presbyterian because I know that there, the seed will fall on fertile soil.

Oh, it's so wonderful Lord, to see what a mite can do. Help me to remember that after You, I am the next one to receive a portion from the bountiful financial blessings You allow me to earn because I am one of your favorite people on earth. Thank you, Lord. AMEN

4/27/04-PRAISE THE LORD! HALLELUJAH!!!

Today I received word that the Dept. of Aging has granted Mother pharmacy money ($400/mo.) for as long as she needs it. This will really be a relief.

5/3/04- MOTHER'S HEART ATTACK

Cat had left a message on my answering service that she had not been able to reach Mother since midnight last night when she got home from giving her a good back scrubbing and helping her into her p.j's. She had tried again at 6 a.m. with no results. I had slept in until 8:30 and tried to call with the same results. I immediately got dressed and had Lee take me over.

When I opened her front door and called to her, she answered and I asked why she hadn't answered her phone. She said she couldn't reach it. I went back to her room and found her lying on the floor. She said she couldn't move her arm because she slept on it all night and asked me to give her a hand to pull her up. I tried but couldn't and then Lee called from downstairs and I asked him to come up.

Mother laughed and I knew that she was thinking about Daddy laughing at the commercial when they say "I've fallen and I can't get up". Mother's chief concern was that I help her find her head rag or put on her wig before Lee came up. We managed to do that together after we tried with my one working arm to get a pillow under her head. Her Life Call button was hanging on the bedroom door.

Lee picked her up and onto the bed and her concern then was that we hurry and get her ready in time to catch the bus to dialysis. Lee asked if she was hurt but she just said her arm was sore from lying on it all night. When Lee helped her into the wheelchair, I got a good look at her face and noticed that her left eye was swollen twice its normal size as well as the side of her face. Her other eye was also swollen and when asked about the fall, she did not remember being on the floor. That's when Lee advised that we call the paramedics.

She was acting so normal otherwise, but

I decided to be safe. That was a wise thing because, upon examination and blood tests at the hospital, it was determined that she had a heart attack with no chest pain. Apparently, the valve in her heart that they had told us was slow to open had been unable to release the blood fast enough that had backed up from the clogged vein to which the shunt was attached. That caused her to pass out but You brought her through. Thank you Lord.

5/9/04- MOTHER'S DAY

We brought Mother home from the hospital yesterday after You performed a miracle on her arm. The doctors were amazed at how quickly her hand and arm had returned to normal after having swollen to the size of a boxing glove. They had explained that it might take several weeks for the blood that had incorporated itself in the tissue to re-enter the bloodstream and reduce the swelling. I guess they forgot that we had You on our side and that makes anything possible.

I am still preparing myself for Mother's pending reunion with You, Daddy, and Mama and am doing my best to add joy to each of the days she has left with us down here. I guess I concentrated on that so much that Mother's Day was somewhat overwhelming. I allowed it to get out of hand, failing to keep the celebration small and limiting it to only close family members. Instead, I allowed people to invite themselves and ended up dead tired with about 45 people here (*lesson learned*). But, since I can't change yesterday, I gave it over to You and went on to enjoy with her the rest of the week that we spent together.

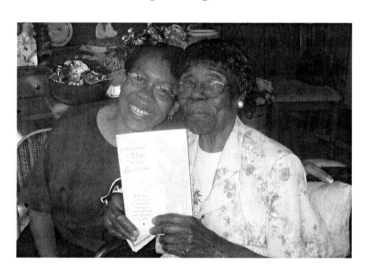

5/11/04 – VACATION FOR 2 AT PARKVIEW

My gift to Mother was our "Home Vacation" and we enjoyed each other immensely at Mother's apartment at Parkview. We had Mother's helper drop us off for her foot appointment and then took a cab to one of our favorite spots to shop—the Goodwill store in Millersville.

Mother was pushing her new *Cadillac* –the walker with the built-in seat and basket she received from Cat, Wayne, and I on Mother's Day. We shopped up and down the aisles with Mother sitting and rolling her walker backwards as we selected beautiful Spring- colored blouses and pants to match. Our favorite dressing room was available and we tried things on and laughed together while we selected the things we loved.

We had smelled the wonderful bread baking at Subway and decided to have lunch there. Mother couldn't chew it very well so we decided to return home to let her finish the soup we had gotten the previous night from our favorite Chinese restaurant. We can make the best out of any situation.

Later that night we had a talk about Mother's options as far as care goes. She still could go to rehab at the Nursing home until she felt stronger or spend her last savings on round-the-clock care, but I knew from the breakdown of my health on Tuesday that I could not do this alone. Cat was unwilling to commit every weekend to staying with her because she needed some time to herself.

Mother prayed on it and came to sit on my bed to talk about it the next morning. She decided to try to make it on her own with the caregivers still coming in 2-3 times each week to help with meals and cleaning. The Physical Therapist was also coming 1-2 times per week. She promised to keep her Life Call button around her neck and try to force feed herself a little more than desired at each meal. We'll just have to leave the rest in Your hands.

Mother, Cat, and I had a great time Sunday after they returned from Church and picked me up to visit Aunt Mamie in the hospital. We took her some flowers from my Mother's Day bush out front and posed with her for some pictures.

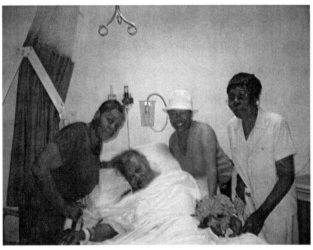

We went to Costco where Mother rode the riding cart and I used her *Cadillac*, purchasing smoothie machines and frozen fruit for both of them. We ended up at another of our favorite spots; Mikie's, where Mother had soup, I sampled several flavors of ice cream, and Cat had a luscious hamburger and fries. What a day! Thank you Lord. AMEN

5/27/04- CCC**

Yesterday, I got word from the accountant that it would be more beneficial to dissolve CCC because we receive no public funding and had been reclassified as a private foundation rather than a tax exempt corporation. It would cost us much more just to file tax statements than we were making. It just doesn't seem like what You would want me to do with the vision You gave me. Instead, You seem to be telling me to "Pass it on".

The first person You brought into my head was the woman we had seen down at Inner Harbor who had come from the Islands and formed a steel drum band made up of the children from St Veronica's Church (the same church that gave CCC the opportunity to teach the Presbyterian kids using their computers).

It's funny how You make all things work together for the good of those who love You.

This woman has done things on her own to train and motivate these kids and gotten grant monies wherever possible to allow her to take them all over to perform. Doesn't this raise their self-esteem, the main goal of CCC? Of course it does and so You are telling me that this is the place to pass the torch and I will. Thank You Lord.

5/30/04

I went to church and sat next to a young lady with braids. Her name is Debbie Kukoyi (we exchanged cards after service). When we were asked to join hands, she took my weak right arm and began to pray in tongues. When she met me at a Mary Kay workshop I had invited her to on the following Thursday, she asked how my affected side was doing. I told her that it was coming along and she said to be patient, the healing would come.

On Friday night when Lee and I went to the movies, my leg felt stronger and I was able to walk with more confidence. Now that I think about it, I have been walking around the house without my brace for most of the week. It is Saturday night - 6/5 - and I walked around and cleaned, cooked, and baked a cake without my brace today. Is there a healing taking place or is this just a fluke? Time will tell but meanwhile, I feel blessed for every moment of strength that You allow. And I'm feeling closer to Lee each day as we work together and play together. Thank You, God. AMEN

6/6/04

I woke up a little after 6 this morning with a feeling of something just not right. Lee was already up checking the water seeping in the basement. I called Mother and made sure all was right with her and then debated whether I was feeling guilty about my decision about not going to church. Then I saw the sparkle in my eyes that always reflects Jesus shining through me and I knew that I would have Him with me wherever I was.

But something is amiss. My critters out back are even acting strange. Those that usually live and eat together are now jumping at each other. I even saw a small rat poke his nose out under the birdfeeder and a squirrel jumped at him. Then another squirrel jumped at a mourning dove, a squirrel climbed *into* the birdfeeder, and Lee went out to chase him away only to find one on the chest where the birdseed is kept. He did not run far even when Lee threw a small stick at him. What is happening? I'm sleepy now even though it is only 10:25 so I think I'll just take a little nap. I'm sure it will all work out.

6/6/04

This morning I got a wake-up call as I reflected back over yesterday. Tracey, Lee's former co-worker came by so that they could go together to the wake of a former co-worker's son. She came in to say Hi and to give me a hug. This morning, I took a look at how I must have looked through her eyes or as Lee could have seen me through other's eyes. I had been dressed in baggy sweatpants and stained sweatshirt all day. I had on socks with my sandals, no makeup, and had not even run a brush through my hair because I still had curls from Friday. I have become so complacent because he shows that he loves me that I don't bother to make myself attractive unless I am planning to go out.

Thanks, God, for the wake-up call. Please help me not to become so comfortable in our relationship that I cease to do that little extra just for him; to put on a little scent and dress in something that will be pleasing to his eye. I know that it is one more way of showing him how much I love him.

6/18/04- Oh Thank You Lord, Hallelujah! You Have Blessed Me Indeed!

So many blessings rained down on me yesterday that I don't want to leave anything out. But I know that it was because I have asked that You blessed me so that I may be a blessing. I just thank you individually for these things:

When I awoke, You led me to call Gwen Bowser to ask if she knew someone who could cook like she does (only healthy) who might be willing to prepare Mother's meals for her. She gave me the name of a friend of hers who, miraculously, lived in Mother's building just one floor below her. She was delighted to take on the task right away and began preparing a delicious pot of homemade soup while we were still talking.

Her name is Leoma (Lee) and she calls herself an old-fashioned Southern cook (just what I have been praying for). She will even plan the meals, shop for the food, prepare it in pureed form, and take it up to Mother. Thank You Jesus! She even offered not to charge for it but, thanks be to God, that You have even made a way to ease that burden. You blessed Mother with the receipt of another settlement check yesterday from one of the companies responsible for Daddy's exposure to asbestos that eventually caused his cancer. You are indeed an *On-time God*. Mother loved the soup and ate a hearty meal of it.

And if that wasn't blessing enough, You had the Christian maintenance lady from one of the schools where I taught return my call and agreed to be one of the models in my "Women Making a Difference" portfolio. I was a little let down when she said that she didn't have many friends that she could share her facial with and, God forgive me, I started to doubt that she might be someone that could benefit me in any way. But You quickly took my mind off of me and reminded me of the spiritual connection we had when we talked at the school. As a reward for my willingness to let You use me, she called a friend who knew the area to bring her out and I suggested that she share the facial and invite some of her friends. She was very receptive of the idea and I found that she works at NSA (a place I used to wok) so we had common ground on which to meet.

You kept on blessing even after that when You encouraged me to take the time to develop a template to record the info from each contact as I spoke with them. That made it much easier to remember what they said to me.

That evening, I went back to my list of ladies I had invited to be my models as far back as 2 yrs ago. That led me to a lady who has her own web design business and works at CSC. She was delighted to come and bring her 2 daughters and the oldest daughter is inviting 2 friends. The Mother has even become excited about coming to our Executive luncheon with our National! When You rain down blessing, You pull out all the stops. How could anyone doubt You?

Because You have shown such faith in me by opening so many doors, I will show my faith in You by not doubting that I can do whatever I need to help these women get what they need. Please give me a listening ear and a receiving heart to hear as well as feel their needs. Help me to remember Your words "Don't force it to be what you want it to be; It will become what it is meant to be; love it; let it flow through you, nurture it; Enjoy the journey." I will Lord and I promise to pass these words along to each lady who joins me on this journey. Thank You. AMEN

8/1/04- Today is Mike's 31st Birthday and I Just Had to Send him this "Love" Gift:

Mike's Birthday Memories (Remember When)

Read Any Good Books…

When you were just 4 years old, I asked what you wanted us to do on your birthday with just the two of us. You said that you wanted us to go somewhere to eat and talk. We drove to the parking lot at Glen Burnie Mall where there was a hot dog truck. We bought hot dogs and drinks, sat on the front seat of the car with your legs sticking straight out because they were too short to reach the floor. When I asked what you might like to talk about, you looked up from your hot dog with a serious look on your little 4-year old face and asked "read any good books lately?" ☺

Birthday Cake With a
4-Wheeler On Top

I think you must have started asking for a 4-wheeler at about age 6. Naturally, as a Mother, my protective spirit did not want you to have one but I had to admire your sense of adventure, always wanting to live on the edge. So, as a way of appeasing us both, I started out early, first with the toy 4—wheeler I put on top of the chocolate birthday cake I baked you. This was my way of saying that I understand your craving but I'll keep you safe beside me for as long as I can. I had not yet grown in Christ enough to realize that He will look out for you in ways I never could. It wasn't until after the motorcycle accident He brought you through that I really acknowledged that I had to let go, and let God. That has been quite a weight lifted from me, especially since your love for speed has only grown since then. I know you keep God extra busy every time you get behind the wheel but He can handle it much better than I. But the next time you feel the need to speed, just remember how

Jamie's last decision is still affecting Bud & Judy. Now I am free to just relax and just enjoy you. Ain't God good? ☺

MEASURING TREE

Remember trampling through the woods over at Dorsey Rd Park on our annual trek to find your measuring tree. We would play "King of the Hill" on our way to find the tree and you would climbed to the highest mound of dirt you could find, pull up all 4 feet of you and stand proudly on top with arms outstretched, and yell "KING OF THE HILL". When we reached the tree, you would back up to it and we would make a mark to see how much you had grown since the previous year. I guess walking through the woods with my 6-year-old could be viewed by others as my version of living on the edge but the woods have been more of a sanctuary for me a place of danger since the time I used to follow my grandfather through them. The smells of fresh dirt and wildflowers, and being able to look

*up through the trees right straight to heaven…
all those were things I wanted to share with you.
And you were willing to follow me anywhere until
some teenage boys walking together through the
woods changed the safe feeling and you looked up at
me and suggested that we might want to look for
another place to continue our birthday tradition.
The depth of your intuition was beginning to show
itself.*

Shopping At Toys 'R Us

*No matter what your choice was for the way we
spent the day, this was the grand finale. You were
allowed to go in and select one item of your choice.
We took our time, playing with toys along the way.
I enjoyed this almost as much as you because I know
that it would have been a dream when I was little
to be allowed to even browse in a toy store. To
actually be able to buy a toy was way beyond the
realm of anything I could have imagined. So now,
I was able to live it through the connection of the*

joy in our spirits. How many parents have that opportunity to have a soul connection with their children and to see the world through their eyes? I'm so glad we do.

LEDO'S

I don't know on which birthday our Ledo's tradition began but it was incorporated as one of the traditions we both wanted to keep. Cold root beer in frosty mugs and a cherry that always wanted to fall to the bottom before we could eat it, and stuffing ourselves with pizza until we couldn't eat another bite. We never ran out of things to talk about. We somehow had a soul connection, always knowing how to make each other laugh.

LYING ON FLAT ROCK

Remember when you were about 10 years old and we decided to go ride bikes on your birthday? We went to the bike path near Litton where I worked and rode daily at lunchtime. After riding side by side and talking, I decided to take you to my favorite spot, the spot where I met with God and felt His peace and left when He quieted my spirit. We went down a small embankment to the edge of a stream where water cascaded between the rocks. Then we stepped from rock to rock until we were out into the stream and onto my favorite flat rock. There, I sat while you lay flat on your back and looked up at the sky as we talked or just kept still while taking in the beauty of the sights and sounds around us. I was reminded once again of what God told me shortly after you were born... that He has great things in store for you. You were created with something buried deep inside you that will enable you to do the great things God created you for. Learn more about God and one day it will be revealed to you what His mission is for you. Meanwhile, Do the part of it you love to do; don't force it to be what you want it to be; it will become what it was meant to be; Love it, let it flow through you, Nurture it; Enjoy the journey.

4-WHEELER DEALER

Not to be forgotten, you reminded me that I said you could have a 4-wheeler when you could afford to buy one. So, now that you had your first BIG job at Little Caesars' pizza (minimum wage AND all the pizza you could eat...every 16-year-old boy's dream job), you wanted to visit the 4-wheeler dealer. So that's exactly what we did. Remember that at one of the dealers, some of the teenage sales guys were releasing mice they had caught onto Ritchie Hwy to see if they could make it across 3 lanes of traffic before being squished. I guess that showed the high caliber of people with whom we were dealing (smile). But it was a change from Toys 'R Us and I began to realize that you had moved into a new phase of your life.

LEXUS & INFINITY

Armed with a new driver's permit, there wasn't much doubt as to where we would spend that birthday. You wanted to go to dealerships and try out these two new cars. You got your first real taste of speed when the Infinity salesman asked you to take it up to 60 and then step on the brake. The car stopped without even jolting us and the look on your face was priceless! (I should know because my eyes were bucked so wide that I could see everything in the car ☺) What an adventure!

So now you are all grown up, 31 years old, married, secure, and into your second new home. God has truly blessed! We're so proud of you and, even though I cannot drive you around right now, I still feel some of that spiritual connection when the two of us get together. Do well, stay tuned to God so as not to miss His plan for you, and never be afraid to step out into untried territory if that is where He leads you. I think that is why He developed that spirit that lets you always feel good about your decisions, so when He gives you the word, there might be no fear or hesitation.

We love you,

Mommy

His reply warmed my heart. It said:

8/2/04

"*Mommy,*

It is too late to call you now, but you can't know how much this means to me. Far better than any gift you could give me, it is this type of memory and heartfelt love that truly grounds me. It allows me to step back and realize the time and love that you and daddy both put into my life that has made Michele and I the people that we are today and allows us to continue to love others as much as you loved us. I consider myself a pretty thankful person and Heather and I will often take time to talk about how blessed we are with our lives to be surrounded by loving families, friends, and each other and this just reiterates that feeling. Thank you very much for sending me this. It is the perfect ending to another wonderful birthday.

Mike"

8/6/04- God is Patient, God is Kind...

God will let you have all the "do overs" you desire until you get it right. Look what He did for the Israelites when He allowed them to take 40 years to get to the place that could have reached in days. I see this morning that He is allowing me to do the same thing. The lessons (building blocks) He has allowed me to learn along the way, I realize that I sometimes forget to use as stepping stones to a get me where he created me to go.

Again, I got so caught up in sharing the info about the business because I knew that He would handle the part I wasn't assigned to do, that I forgot the lessons I had learned about earning and managing money so I could benefit and pass that lesson on to those who followed me. Lord, forgive me and thank you for your patience. Thank you for dropping reminders in my spirit during the time I meditate with you. I will begin to work on this today.

I am going to the Dr this morning concerning bruises that I have noticed appearing on my body since March, or maybe longer. Please let it be something that can easily be cured and give the Dr the wisdom to diagnose it correctly. Whatever your will, please help me to be able to accept it and live with it. AMEN

FOLLOW UP:

The Dr found that bruising is one of the side effects of taking Plavix, a stroke prevention medicine. We agreed that the medicine's benefits far outweigh the side effects. Thank you Lord for the simple answer to my concern.

8/13/04- Isn't God Wonderful?

Yesterday, for the first time in my 60 years of life, I came eye to eye with a hummingbird. I was sitting in my favorite place—the swing in my prayer garden, having a sandwich of fresh tomatoes from my vine, when out of the corner of my eye, I saw movement. There, sipping nectar from the beautiful pink flowers not 2 feet from me was a beautiful gray hummingbird with a black- tipped tail, beak and eyes. He hovered right there long enough for me to appreciate his beauty and then flitted away up to the flowers in the hanging pots on the deck. Thank you, Father, for the little serendipitous events you sprinkle into my life to make each day just a little more special.

In briefly reading back over this journal, I

noticed that I forgot to mention the backyard swing we got. I have always wanted one because for some reason, it reminds me of Mama's (Mother's Mother) house though I can't really remember a porch swing there. Cat, Mother, and I were at Costco one day and saw this fabulous swing and knew we had to have it. Cat and I both bought one. It has a beautiful carved arch on top of it's heavy metal stand and a fringed canopy that Lee angled just right so that I can sit in shade no matter what the sun's angle may be.

It also captures whatever breezes come along to cool me under the trees. I am so blessed! I take my smoothie or my lunch out there along with my phone and whatever work I need to do, and I can commune with You, enjoy my critters, and accomplish whatever is needed at the same time. I am also blessed with a tomato plant that is even more fabulous than the one last year, yielding big, sweet tomatoes that weigh nearly half a pound each and growing 2-3 on each stem. Lee also planted grape tomatoes that I pluck and eat warm right off the vine. Life is good!

Cat, Rita, and I enjoyed our trip to the spa so much last week that Cat and I have booked another in September to include Mother and Hattie. Cat is blooming before our eyes, learning to pamper herself and leaving things in Your hands that she used to worry about. We can see the glow on her face and she is looking happier than I can remember her looking in her life. Thank you, God. AMEN

9/30/04- JOYCE'S MANSION

Last night, I was blessed to take 3 of my best Mary Kay people to an evening at Joyce's Million-dollar mansion. What an inspirational evening! One lady who was most instrumental in helping me to earn my first Mary Kay car and there to celebrate the earning of my second, came as she said she would. I never knew until You inspired Joyce to talk about her worse day in Mary Kay (the day she thought she had earned her first Cadillac and she missed by not tracking the numbers) that my friend quit doing Mary Kay for the same reason.

Another wonderful angel you brought to cross my path was Jackie who had told me earlier this week that she had read the material I gave her and she knew that she had no desire to do this. Yet you had her call 20 minutes before we were to leave and tell me that she was on her way. What a blessing! After seeing and listening to Joyce, she is sure that she now wants to do it. Thank You Lord.

And for Michele, who took the step that allowed me and the others to get the chance to attend this event because I needed a recruit in order to earn the right to go. Michele has decided that this time she will really put effort into her business because she now sees the bigger picture. Bless us Lord.

You told me that all I have is all I need to accomplish the purpose for which You put me here, so I'll no longer wait until my body heals more. You have shown me that there are people around who willingly help shore me up where I am weak and You let me help them in areas where I am strong. Again I thank You.

Joyce has told me that I have 3 units within my client base already. She has asked me to pick my sharpest (mentally, spiritually, and with good work ethics) to ask to walk this journey with me. This morning You gave me 18 names.

I see Your hand in the plan and hear Your voice saying "Trust and Believe". Just when I was beginning to wonder if my labors were in vain, You are showing me that the seeds I planted will bear fruit in Your time. Thank You Lord for the reinforcement of my belief and for Lee, Loretta, and Joyce who never stopped believing in me. AMEN

10/19/04

So much has happened recently that I haven't taken time to write for a while but today I've been urged to make an entry. It's as if the Lord said "Write". In reading my Daily Guideposts entry this morning, I was again reminded to "Do the part of it I love to do…". It seems that I can write easily and well about plans and experiences but following through with the plans with consistently is a weakness. Could it be that He endowed me with the ability to write and wants me to use it or am I going out on a tangent again? I will look into the publishing of my journals again and see where that leads me.

Meanwhile, God has blessed us to keep the circle unbroken for yet another day. Cat is in the hospital again for what is perhaps the 10th time or more within a month's time. They cannot seem to discover what is making fluid gather in her body, around her lungs and heart making it hard for her to breathe and her chest to hurt. Please cure her Lord if it be Your will. We put her into Your loving hands.

Thank You also for the portion of health You have allowed Mother and for allowing her, Cat, and me to attend Aunt Mamie's 90th birthday party last Saturday night. Thank You for Thelma who worked tirelessly to make sure that it was a memorable event, including a trip for Aunt Mamie to get her hair and nails done and be picked up in a limo. Thank You for blessing me to be able to videotape the party because Lee had a wedding to do on Eastern Shore. Aunt Mamie even danced, with help, and spoke. It was a blessed event. Mother and I had to take a cab there but You provided us with a really nice driver. Thank You.

Our home is in a bit of disarray because we are having the long-awaited bathroom renovation done on a grand scale which includes a room with a shower, sink and a Jacuzzi with a half wall separating them. The toilet is enclosed in a small room with a window. Lee had selected a beautifully carved wood vanity with a marble-topped sink to go into the room with the Jacuzzi and we both loved the smaller wooden mirrored vanity he had seen with a matching stool. We selected a mirror to be placed over the sink and plan to go back to Pennsylvania to pick up the painting we both fell in love with when we saw it at the Colorfest we took the boys to while camping last week.

The best thing about this project Lord is that we are incorporating ideas from both of us and making it a room we really love. Thank You for the experience. I'm so glad You delayed our building it when I thought I wanted it years ago. It would not have been so rich an experience as it is now. They say that Your delay is not Your denial and I'm sure that You mean for me to apply this bit of wisdom to other situations in my life as well.

Thank You for this talk this morning and I can't finish this without thanking You once again for Lee who brought order out of the chaos that the building process left, making the house uninhabitable so that we had to stay somewhere else for a few days. Thank You for Mike and Heather opening up their new home and welcoming us to stay for 3 nights with them. You have surrounded me with love and made me know once again that I am special in Your sight. Help me to pass that love on Lord. Bless me that I may be a blessing to others. AMEN

10/20/04

This morning, I was given a gentle push to get me back "on purpose". In my morning reading, I was reminded that we're all made with talent to do different things and we should recognize and give over to someone else the things we *weren't* created for. Again the words "*Do the part of it you love to do*" echoed in my mind. I had stopped offering ladies the Mary Kay opportunity because I felt guilty about not following through with them; pestering them until they signed up to be a Beauty Consultant, set up their Open House, and ordered. Again I found myself bugging them about parts of this business that made me uncomfortable; areas better left to others. But after You had me review what I had written when You started me on this latest mission, I realized that I had let other well-meaning people make me feel guilty about not doing all portions of the process. Therefore, I stopped doing any of it.

Lord, help me to stick to my guns, doing the part I feel good about and releasing the guilt to You when others try to steer me the way they think best. Thank you for Jean DeVeaux whose soul made a connection with mine as I felt the passion in her about working to improve women's lives. I was perfectly content not to try to persuade her to do what I do but to work with her to find if Mary Kay might be the answer to other women's prayers.

You are growing me, God, to see beyond this little box that I have kept myself in. Thank You. And I think that, for awhile, until I grow stronger and more resolute, I will communicate my ideas to Loretta mainly by email lest I be influenced to stray from my purpose. Help me, God, to stay on purpose and to word the letter I will send to her in a way that helps her to understand. I really feel that we can each use our strengths to carry out this mission. AMEN

10/21/04

Good Morning Lord. Thank You for waking me just in time to listen to the "Spiritual Vitamin" on the radio. It inspired me to once again pull out my special copy of the Bible and I found myself looking back over the passages I had marked, the picture of Mother standing under Daddy's picture, and the copy of the Prayer of Jabez given to me by Neet, another Mary Kay Consultant close to my heart.

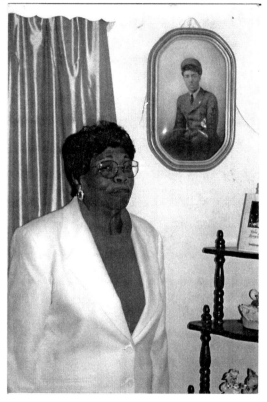

Today's Spiritual Vitamin reminded me to follow closely in Your footsteps, staying as close to You as I can get. That way, I know that my way is safe and I will go where You want me to go. I will listen and with Your help, try harder not to be distracted and drawn away.

I sent the letter to Loretta. It read as follows:

10/20/04

Dear Loretta,

Again, I find my progress at a standstill and my joy at this task waning. I believe that I have gone "off purpose" and I think I know the reason why. I have failed to follow God's directive to **"do the part of it you love to do"**. *After having wonderful facials with the women I met and sending them home with information, I was once again feeling trapped into bugging them to overcome objections, schedule an Open House (which you might remember I always hated to do myself), and to order inventory. Of course I know that these are all necessary parts of getting started in this business but they are not my strengths. You, on the other hand, appear strong in these areas but I have felt guilty about having you do all the hard work while I get the commission.*

These are the tasks I think are involved in getting others started in this business. I enjoy doing items 1, 2, 3(with you), & 7-9.

1) Facial – intro info

2) Glamour – 2nd info

3) Lunch, coffee, or conference call – decision

4) Follow-up

5) Inventory decision

6) Setup Open House

7) Do Open House

8) Invite to 1st month's training

9) Inform of special events

10) Remind of order time and status

If we can agree that someone else will do the others and that the subject of Directorship will be dropped until it evolves, I think I can get back on purpose. Meanwhile, I think that communication by email will work best for me because it gives me a chance to think through what I want to communicate and allows me not to be pulled off my course by your magnetic personality. Together, we can make this work.

Love, Cecelia

Loretta replied that same night, even after being out all day driving around to do training at 2 distant places. She agreed to work with me in the ways that I suggested and again released me from the things that were uncomfortable for me. Thank You for her understanding and patient spirit Lord. She is truly setting the example of what a Leader should be and I know that I will take over the weak areas as I regain confidence. I once passed on words to her from You that I thought were meant for her—"Struggling Directors produce struggling Directors". Perhaps the message was meant for me. Thank You Lord. AMEN

10/22/04- DADDY'S BIRTHDAY

He would have been 83 today. I called to remind Mother of it today and tell her that I would be spending tonight and tomorrow with her in celebration. She was happy about that but said that she had forgotten his birthday. Because it has rained for the past 2 days, I think that it may be too muddy to go to the gravesite but just being with her will make her happy. Cat will be invited to join us for as much of the time as she would like but her health has been bad for more than 3 months now so I don't know if she can come. If she does, I think we will go to see T.D. Jakes' movie "Woman Thou Art Loosed".

Mother's friend, Lee is sick and so we'll be on our own for meals but we'll do all right. My Lee will be doing weddings tonight and tomorrow so this works out just fine, allowing Scott & crew to work undisturbed on the bathroom. You always work things out. Thank You. AMEN

This has been a month of significant blessings so I decided to type instead of write. Thank you, Lord for bringing Mother through her many trips to the emergency room by ambulance because of real pain that the doctors have not been able to diagnose, only lessen with medication. Thanks for blessing me with the ability to stay overnight on a number of occasions, no longer feeling disapproval from Lee for putting my health in harms way. Thank you for helping him to understand.

Thanks, also, for the joy Mother and I shared as we went to sleep whenever we felt like it and sometimes got up at 2a.m. to eat soup and dessert together or take showers where she got her back scrubbed and lotioned. The freedom we felt as we walked undressed from bathroom to bedrooms, she without her wig and me in just my "Hawaiian" skin (she always said that my skin color was like that of the guy we took pictures with when we went to Hawaii).

Thanks for the time we took a cab together on a beautiful day You sent and went to Wal-Mart where we both drove the carts around and shopped. What fun to feel the freedom to get around again. Had it not been for the stroke, I would not have truly known what freedom she was feeling. The absolute greatest blessing for her came at the end of the month after we had gone through a series of unreliable caregivers and Mother was growing weaker and in need of more care. We had even gotten to the point where I had sent for information on assisted living facilities which we both dreaded.

Then You stepped in right on time and had her new best friend, Lee, hurt her back and become unable to do the heavy lifting required at her nursing job. She asked Mother if we would consider having her be Mother's helper 7 days a week doing the things that she was already doing better than those who were paid to do it. She will continue to prepare all of Mother's meals, shop for her food, and do her laundry. She would even take Mother with her when she wants to go. And she is doing all of this for $300/week, just a little over the amount we were paying for the caregiver to come for only 3 hours/day 3 times/week. Hallelujah! You are an On-time God.

Thank you also for answering our prayers to bring Cat safely through surgery to remove her gallbladder. She drove herself to the emergency room down here after being in constant pain and going to Sinai ~20 times in the past 2 months with no results. The doctors say that this surgery might not solve all of her problems because she is also suffering severe headaches on the right side and fluid build up causing difficulty breathing. But they tried to resolve one problem at a time. Byron moved out of Cat's house yesterday and in with his new girlfriend, Sonjia. I pray that he has made a wise decision.

Lee's cousin, Queen, died suddenly, on

the last day of the month with a heart attack. Thank you for strengthening the family as they go through this.

Lee and I have grown closer still as we enjoy visiting antique shops and different stores, together selecting different items for our new customized bathroom. It is wonderful watching it come together. Thank you for the inspiration to ask Scott about using his restaurant for Lee's 60th birthday party. I'm excited about making it a memorable occasion and to give back to Lee some of the joy he has given to others. Bless our efforts, Lord. AMEN

11/4/04- TRANSFER OF POWER

For the past couple of months, I have felt twinges in my left (good) foot, which have forced me to put more weight on my right. Now, I have started therapy to help heal the tendon I sprained in the good foot. When it appeared that I no longer have "a leg to stand on", You have given me the wisdom to step back to see the good that You are allowing me to accomplish with this latest challenge. I can see the "transfer of power" back to the side You originally made stronger. Now, every time I feel the pain, I try to use that as a reminder to put the weight back where it belongs.

Thank you God for wisdom and for Lee who steps in when I can stand no longer and helps me complete whatever task I have undertaken. He brings my drink into the living room after

I carry in the plate, brings the laundry up from downstairs after I have finished it, and waits patiently after the movie for me to get my legs and feet moving again. He is such a blessing. AMEN

11/5/04- ROBERT'S APPENDIX

Thank You God for Cat's strength as she recovers from her gall bladder operation only one week ago and is now at the hospital with Robert. The doctors thought last night that he may have to have surgery but I don't know if that has taken place. Thank You for keeping Cat's heart and mind while she deals with each new challenge and still deals with the grief of losing Cliff. Bless me Lord and strengthen me so that I may continue to be a blessing to those who need me.

I feel a little more strength and balance today and my tendon feels a little better. Negative thoughts keep trying to tell me that I'm not doing things as well as I was doing them a year ago when I was closer to the stroke date but I know that You are strengthening me as much as is needed to enable me to accomplish what You would have me do. Keep upmost in my mind, Lord, that I only need to do the part of it I love to do and not be concerned with the outcome.

My concern over the end result, and what appears to be a lack of progress toward the goal that friends and compatriots have set for me, sometimes causes me to stop in my tracks and accomplish less than my best. I will refocus on the goals You set for me and I thank You for the reminder.

As I looked up from typing, You just showed me hundreds of birds all following one leader. That leader is a symbol of me and I know that I will just need to post reminders of my progress and look at them daily. Thank You Lord. AMEN – (I'm looking out at beautiful orange streaks You are painting across the sky. What a wonderful artist You are!)

11/15

My first thoughts this morning were feelings of love and gratitude as I looked over at Lee's peaceful, sleeping face. At times like that, I want to reach over and kiss him softly on his beautiful lips but I don't want to disturb his rest because, once he wakes up, he will be in action all day, providing for the needs of everyone (especially me). Thank You God for his love.

I showered this morning in our new shower in our room built with love. It was so warm and relaxing as I sat on the built-in seat that I didn't want it to end. After stepping out into the warm air blowing from the overhead heater, I really felt luxurious. I had to call Lee initially because I could not close the shower door that Scott gerry-rigged until he has the other part of the door custom cut. Then I had to call him again because I couldn't get the door open. But it was wonderful in between. I regret that Lee didn't have Scott exchange the door for one he really wanted but Lee hates to bother people, so he settled for this one.

This bathroom is truly one we built with love and I can feel God's presence in there especially as I sit on the wide chair under the skylight. I truly feel that God allows me these little pieces of luxury to let me know that I don't have to do what others think I should do in order to have the riches that make Lee and me happy. This room would not mean nearly as much if we had a decorator design it because it would not have the loving memories built in—memories of Lee and I shopping and selecting pieces together. Thank You God.

The phone in the water closet rang while I was still in reverie. It was Mother calling to say that Cat had been re-admitted to the hospital out here with stomach pains, fluid build up, and shortness of breath. Please help her Lord. I give her over to You. You told me to have Thelma contact the Head of Surgery to see her. I left a message for her and told her the message came from You. I know that You will give him the wisdom to work on her problem, and with

Your help, to solve it. Thank You.

I have an appointment to see my Primary Care Physician to get a referral for me to get the therapy I need to complete the transition of power back to my dominant (right) side. Thank you for letting that come to pass. AMEN

11/27/04

Thank you God for this beautiful, blue-skied, sunny day. Outside, it is probably in the 40's, but we are cozy and warm in here. Thank you for letting us see one more Thanksgiving with Mother still here with us. You have even been gracious enough to let her walk with help into Michele's house to share the joy and fellowship of another dinner together.

She took her friend and helper, Leoma (Lee) to Lee's 60th birthday party that was held at Scott's restaurant (Ambrosia's) in Cherry Hill. All the brothers and sisters (except Linda, who is in Taiwan and Sandra, who hardly attends any family function since her bout with breast cancer) were there and we had a great time. Even Gwen was back up here from North Carolina and was able to come. There were more than 40 guests, including:

Michele, Everett, Cameron, Ethan, Mike, Heather, Jay, Weldon, Paula, Nece, Sharon, Virginia, Becky, Ellen, Richard, Raheem, Charles, Little Charles, Little Weldon, Taurus, Taurus's friend, Francine, Reatha, Aunt Liz, Mother, Leoma, Cat, Rita, Keren, Shirley, Gene, Martina, Gerald, Thelma, Jerome, Danny, Vernetta, Gwen Bowser, Paula's sister, Sharon, and I.

Michele had the cake made at B.J's with pictures on top that showed Lee when he was a baby and then the picture taken last year when Mike took him down on the field at Raven's stadium.

I thank you, God, for the birthday grace so lovingly prayed by Ellen and the Thanksgiving prayer read by Cameron. I had regrets about not praying my earnest prayer of thanks out loud, thanking You for the special love You've allowed me to receive from the two people whose hands I held during the Thanksgiving prayer, Lee's & Mother's. No greater love could I receive than from the two of them You have surrounded me with down here. Thank you, Lord.

Thanks also for the love and fun shared with Lee as we prepared 2 turkeys for the Thanksgiving feast from a recipe he saw demonstrated on TV. Preparation was as much fun as eating it as we got up that morning, chopped and sautéed onions and celery, made it into stuffing, and separated the skin from the breast to allow us to insert stuffing under the skin. We even poked hole in the legs and inserted smoky bacon, fresh rosemary, and garlic. We stuffed rosemary and a large, microwaved naval orange inside the bird and I was given the pleasure of giving the turkey a massage with olive oil sprinkled with salt and pepper. It was so pretty that I took a picture of it. (Mike said later that it looked painful).

I roasted one in the oven while Lee put

the other on the grill. Then, after traditionally watching the end of the Macy's Thanksgiving Day Parade, I kicked back in the recliner and snuggled in for a peaceful nap. You even kept the ankle pain away long enough for me to accomplish all of that. Thank you, Lord, for such a blessed life.

This morning, Ms. Bell (Uncle Ernest's second wife is being funeralized. I had said that I wasn't going because it would require me to have someone carry and push my wheelchair as well as look out for Mother and her walker. When I awoke this morning, however, I decided to ask Lee to go and take us because it might be the last time Mother got to see some of those people attending. He said "No" (a rarity for him). Thank You for letting me accept that without anger. I know that even You say "No" to me sometime and I'm one of Your favorite people. So, for whatever reason he thought he gave me that answer, I know that he is being directed by You and I thank You for letting him be an instrument for Your love. AMEN

11/30

The last day of November and I just sat in the new water closet, looking at the sky and counting how many ways You have blessed me. Mother is still down here walking with us another hour into our journey. Cat is seeking the wisdom and courage to let her full-time job become part time. You have lessened the pain in my leg and I can start to exercise it more. Lee is still peacefully sleeping giving me unhurried time with You. The kids and grandkids are all loving us and each other...so many blessings that I cannot count them all. Thank You Lord.

I keep thinking of things that I could have (should have) expressed out loud to the people gathered at the birthday party and at Thanksgiving; things like my statement that Lee is living proof that I have found favor with You because You chose someone so loving and supportive to walk this journey with me. I wanted to tell all of his loved ones not to worry about him *finding You* because You have truly *found him* and those who really know him can see You shining through him in all his acts of love. But again, You have assured me that it was not necessary to say it, but to know it, and give thanks for it. Sometimes, I am amazed at the wisdom You are giving me. Again, I thank You, Lord. AMEN

12/10- Our Serenity Room

It's almost done, 2 months after the work began and about 4 months after the plans were hatched. It became a living thing; full of changes as Lee and I discovered a piece at an antique store, a markdown warehouse, and an expensive tile store…each piece is wrapped in memories. Thank you, God.

We chose the color, a serene green; based on a picture I saved from a magazine and ultimately fell in love with in Mike's new home. It was initially going to be just an update to our old bathroom, but love had it evolve into a room where God dwells.

It has an entry door that connects it with our bedroom so, in the Spring, we can open it, the window at the front of the house, and the French doors leading into the sunroom and have air and sunshine flow gently through this entire wing. As you enter the room from our bedroom, to your right, standing on an easel, is a full-length mirror with a dark wood-like frame and a scroll on top. Beside that is the entryway to our water (Prayer) closet that contains a toilet and a sink we selected together from the "Door Store" where a man had a "Door Dog", a large, old German Shepherd that quietly followed the man everywhere he went.

There is also a small window in there that greets me with the beautiful orange and blue streaked sky that signals the start of a new day. This is where I meet with God to thank him for taking us safely through the night and where I read the message He has for me in my "Daily Guidepost" book.

The floor in 2/3 of the room is covered with a heavy marble tile. Next to the prayer closet is our shower with a built-in little seat, a showerhead that can be slid to different positions on a pole, and a large showerhead (a surprise from Lee) that sprays water that feels like drops of rain on your skin. I keep the mango-fragranced bath gel on the soap dish in there. I got that as a gift when Lee and I stopped in the Bath & Body Shop before our movie started on one of our Date Nights.

There is an extra-wide comfortable chair, with a wooden curved back and a padded cushion in front of a half wall. On top of the wall, suspended from the ceiling, will be the most beautiful double-paned stained glass window, one that Lee and I discovered at an antique store. We both instantly fell in love with it and knew that it had to be a part of that room. Scott is framing it and, along with the vanity mirror that Scott is having custom cut, and it will be the final piece that he will contribute to the room.

On either side of the stained glass wall will be plants that Lee so lovingly nurture. There is a skylight that spills light and the sounds of raindrops on the roof when it rains. You can sit in the chair, look up to the heavens, and almost feel God's love flowing down. I am hoping that

Lee will suspend the stained glass angel from the skylight so that the sun can shine through her. It will be as though angels are descending straight from Heaven to watch over us.

Lee professionally installed speakers, flush with the ceiling to provide beautiful music while I wash, bathe, or meditate. Who knew God had added that to Lee's list of talents?

On the other side of the wall is an elegant piece that is the focal point of the entire room. It is a richly-carved walnut cabinet with curved front and legs, 8 small drawers with antique-looking brass handles, and a center door. It has a marble top in which sits a sink. The entire room was designed around this piece that Lee saw, loved, and took me to see before plans were even in place. Over the sink hangs a mirror, framed with scrollwork and coordinating magnificently with the cabinet. Live plants add to the beauty.

There is a window in which sits a small blown-glass statue of a Mother and baby dolphin leaping out of a wave. We found that at the Applefest/Colorfest where we took the boys camping this summer. Under the window is the Jacuzzi, a joy to use as it massages my muscles and gives comfort to my aching joints, surrounding me with wonderful fragrances that make me feel luxurious.

The whole feeling of this room is summed up in the picture that hangs there that shows Lee's flower garden blooming in full color in November 2004.

This room was created from
Love
GOD is here

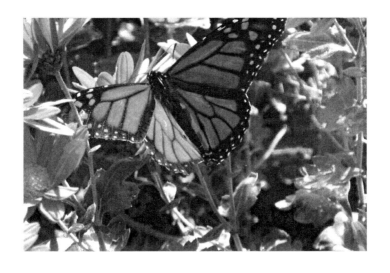

Lee's flower garden

November 2004

12/9/04

I am about to go through a major transition in my life, one in which I let God flow through me without blocking my blessings. I'm not sure what it is but I know that, as long as He is with me and allows Lee to continue this journey with me, I shall be happy. I see and feel the changes about to take place as God brings me into my season. Bless me Lord and allow me to be a blessing to all whose path I cross during this phase of my journey. Transition is scary but exciting. Help me remember that You did not give me the spirit of fear and that I can do ALL things through Christ who strengthens me. AMEN

Breinigsville, PA USA
26 August 2009
222971BV00001B/2/P